Essential Reports
for
Anaesthetists

Essential Reports
for
Anaesthetists

P. R. Hambly

Nuffield Department of Anaesthesia
John Radcliffe Hospital
Oxford, UK

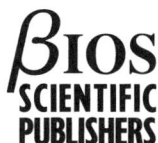

βIOS
SCIENTIFIC
PUBLISHERS

© BIOS Scientific Publishers Limited, 1997

First published 1997

A CIP catalogue record for this book is available from the British Library.

ISBN 1 859962 11 4

BIOS Scientific Publishers Ltd
9 Newtec Place, Magdalen Road, Oxford OX4 1RE, UK
Tel. +44 (0) 1865 726286. Fax +44 (0) 1865 246823
World Wide Web home page: http://www.Bookshop.co.uk/BIOS/

DISTRIBUTORS

Australia and New Zealand
Blackwell Science Asia
54 University Street
Carlton, South Victoria 3053

India
Viva Books Private Limited
4325/3 Ansari Road, Daryaganj
New Delhi 110002

Singapore and South East Asia
Toppan Company (S) PTE Ltd
38 Liu Fang Road, Jurong
Singapore 2262

USA and Canada
BIOS Scientific Publishers
PO Box 605, Herndon
VA 20172-0605

Important Note from the Publisher
The information contained within this book was obtained by BIOS Scientific Publishers Ltd from sources believed by us to be reliable. However, while every effort has been made to ensure its accuracy, no responsibility for loss or injury whatsoever occasioned to any person acting or refraining from action as a result of information contained herein can be accepted by the authors or publishers.

The reader should remember that medicine is a constantly evolving science and while the authors and publishers have ensured that all dosages, applications and practices are based on current indications, there may be specific practices which differ between communities. You should always follow the guidelines laid down by the manufacturers of specific products and the relevant authorities in the country in which you are practising.

Typeset by Creative Associates, Oxford, UK.
Printed by Biddles Ltd, Guildford, UK.

Contents

Clinical guidelines

CONTENTS

Personnel, workload, hours

Organization

NHS

Audits

Training and education

Contents

A&E	Accident and Emergency
AAC	Advisory Appointments Committee
ACMT	Advisory Committee on Medical Training
ACTS	Advisory Committee on Toxic Substances
ADA	anaesthetic department assistant
ADN	anaesthetic department nurse
AIDS	acquired immunedeficiency syndrome
ARDS	adult respiratory distress syndrome
BMA	British Medical Association
BMI	body mass index
CCST	Certificate of Completion of Specialist Training
CDS	Community Dental Services
CEPOD	Confidential Enquiry into Perioperative Deaths
CHC	Community Health Council
CME	continuing medical education
CNS	central nervous system
COAD	chronic obstructive airways disease
COSHH	Control of Substances Hazardous to Health
CPR	cardiopulmonary resuscitation
CRDC	Central Research and Development Committee
CSF	cerebrospinal fluid
CVP	central venous pressure
DoH	Department of Health
DSU	day surgery unit
ECG	electrocardiogram
ECT	electroconvulsive therapy
FHSA	Family Health Service Authority
FRCA	Fellowship of The Royal College of Anaesthetists
GDP	general dental practitioner
GDS	General Dental Services
GMC	General Medical Council
GP	general practitioner
HBV	hepatitis B virus

HDS	Hospital Dental Services
HDU	High Dependency Unit
HIV	human immunodeficiency virus
HST	higher specialist training
HTM	Health Technical Memorandum
ICU	Intensive Care Unit
INR	International Normalised Ratio
ITU	Intensive Therapy Unit
IVRA	intravenous regional anaethesia
NCVQ	National Council for Vocational Qualifications
NHD	national half-day
NTN	national training number
NVQ	National Vocational Qualification
ODA	operating department assistant
ODP	operating department practitioners
OES	occupational exposure standard
R&D	Research and Development
RAST	radioallergosorbent
RCA	Royal College of Anaesthetists
RCM	Royal College of Midwives
RDRD	Regional Offices' Director of R&D
SIFTR	Service Increment for Teaching and Research
WLI	waiting list initiative
WTE	whole-time equivalent

This book contains the key points of 69 Working Party reports and other documents that are of interest to anaesthetists in a clinical or professional sense.

The book is intended to serve many functions, none of which is to remove the need to read the original reports. This collection is, I hope, fairly comprehensive. The list of contents is thus a reference work in itself, which can be used by those new to the speciality and others to identify documents that they need to read. The index provides a rapid mechanism to search the current official guidance on any individual topic, or to find official definitions. This may assist in the design of audit projects and such like. The précised reports act as a quick reference to the key findings, and provide information on how to obtain a copy of the original. The section on further reading provides a list of documents that are of historical or more minority interest. Again, details of how to obtain them are supplied. Finally, I have enclosed a complete list of 'Safety Action Bulletins' that have relevance to anaesthesia. I hope this will find a useful place on the shelves of new trainees, examination candidates, interviewees and others.

The reports are presented in précis form, and I have stripped each down to the minimum relevant information. This means that you are at the mercy of my idea of 'minimum' and 'relevant'. Where a particular report gives a summary, this is reproduced verbatim, and shown in italic text. Words such as 'currently', 'yet' or 'at present' mean **'at the time of original publication'**. The publication date is supplied where this is provided on the original.

I have made every effort to convey accurately the main points of each report. However, anyone planning serious decisions, or wishing to make direct quotes should **refer to the original document**. This book is intended to summarise key principles and we cannot accept responsibility for erroneous impressions gained through not reading the original.

It seems that none of us is immune from occasional spelling errors, split infinitives, inappropriate plural verbs, and transmutal gerunditives and, where these occur, I have generally tidied them up, but not always in passages reproduced 'verbatim'. Errors in other passages are all my own work. (OK, I made up 'transmutal gerunditives'). Much confusion and inconsistency exists about words like 'vaporizer' and 'analyser', which should be spelt thus.

Should this project prove useful, I hope it will be able to evolve further with future editions, and to this end constructive suggestions on style, format, and what to include or omit are welcome, particularly by e-mail: prhambly@globalnet.co.uk.

P. R. Hambly

Day Case Surgery:
The Anaesthetist's Role in Promoting High Quality Care

Clinical and organisational guidelines for safe provision of day surgery services.

INTRODUCTION

The provision of day surgery requires meticulous preoperative preparation, close liaison with community services and specialised perioperative care by staff trained in day surgery.

The purpose-built self-contained unit is the ideal, but the practice of admitting patients to a day unit and operating on them in main theatres on a day case list can also produce high quality care. Mixing day-stay patient with in-patients in wards or on lists is less satisfactory.

Day surgery needs a co-ordinated approach, and must be audited.

SELECTION OF PATIENTS

There are no absolute criteria of fitness for day surgery.

Assessment falls into four categories: social, medical, facility, personnel.

Social factors
- The patient must be willing to undergo day surgery.
- There must be a responsible adult able and willing to care for the patient at home for at least the first 24 hours.
- Patients or their carers should have access to a telephone.
- The home situation should be compatible with postoperative care, that is have adequate heating, lighting, kitchen, bathroom and toilet facilities.

Medical factors
- The patient or carer should understand the procedure and subsequent postoperative care.
- The patient should be fully fit or with well controlled chronic illness.
- The patient's Quetlet ratio [$=wt(kg) \div ht(m)^2$] should be less than 30.
- Patients should be assessed fully before admission for the procedure, appropriate investigations ordered and informed consent obtained.
- Patients should be selected according to their physiological status not their age.

Published in February 1994 by The Association of Anaesthetists of Great Britain and Ireland.

Facility factors
- Care should be provided in a facility set aside for day surgery.
- Simple, rapid and effective exchange of information should be possible between hospital and community personnel.
- Information technology should be provided to enable audit to take place.
- Day stay patients currently treated in specialised units (e.g. ophthalmology, psychiatry) need not necessarily be managed in a centralised unit, provided that the same standards of assessment, care and follow up are provided.

Personnel factors
- Care should be consultant-led.
- Nurses and other staff should be specially trained and allocated to day surgery.
- General practitioners (GPs) and other community staff must agree that the patient can receive this kind of care, and should be able to visit the day surgery unit (DSU).

DOCUMENTATION

Examples of assessment forms are available from the British Association of Day Surgery.

Information booklets should also be produced, explaining the day care process. Specific information sheets relevant to the individual procedures should also be given to the patient.

STAFFING

Each DSU should have a medical director. A consultant anaesthetist with management experience is ideally suited to such a post.

Each unit should also have adequate staffing, led by a senior nurse, as well as reception staff and operating department practitioners (ODPs). Each unit should formulate its own staffing structure according to local needs.

Each unit should have a management group, comprising representatives of all interested parties, which should write operational policies, organise marketing and audit.

ANAESTHETIC MANAGEMENT

Anaesthetic techniques should aim to minimise stress, maximise comfort and prevent morbidity such as nausea and vomiting. Analgesia is paramount and must be long lasting. Standards of monitoring and assistance should be the same as for in-patient procedures.

RECOVERY

Anaesthetic techniques for day surgery should ensure rapid recovery. Standards of postoperative supervision must be as high as for in-patients.

DISCHARGE

Patients must fulfil established discharge criteria before they leave the DSU. Every patient must be seen postoperatively by both surgeon and anaesthetist. Assessment of 'street fitness' can be made by nursing staff, according to the unit's written policy.

There must be access to in-patients for patient beds with postoperative complications.

DISCHARGE FOLLOWING REGIONAL ANAESTHESIA

Residual neural blockade after spinal or epidural anaesthesia may cause postural hypotension and urinary retention despite return of motor and sensory function. Pflug *et al.* (1978) have suggested four criteria to be met before discharge.

1. Return of sensation in perianal area.
2. Plantar flexion of the foot (while supine) at the same strength as that prior to anaesthesia.
3. Return of proprioception in the big toe.
4. The patient is not sedated or hypovolaemic.

The ability to evert the foot demonstrates return of S1 motor function, and indicates that the patient will be able to walk safely. This may avoid the need for testing perianal sensation.

Patients may be discharged with residual sensory or motor block after peripheral nerve blocks and intravenous regional anaesthesia. They must be given adequate information.

POSTOPERATIVE INSTRUCTIONS

All patients should receive verbal and written instructions on discharge. These should:

- warn of symptoms they may experience;
- advise against driving, drinking alcohol, operating machinery or cooking;
- give guidance about removal of sutures, etc.;
- give a list of contact telephone numbers for use in the event of a problem.

DISCHARGE SUMMARY

The patient's GP should be informed, by phone or fax, of the operation, the anaesthetic and the patient's discharge.

CONTRACTUAL ARRANGEMENTS

Day unit sessions should be designated as fixed commitments in an anaesthetist's job plan. Time for pre- and postoperative assessment should be included as part of the flexible sessions.

THE FUTURE

The provision of day surgery will increase in the future. There will be new operations, improved anaesthetic techniques and increased use of regional anaesthesia. Hotel facilities will be built close to DSUs.

Day Surgery: Making it Happen

Identifies the benefits of day surgery and makes recommendations for its development.

SYNOPSIS

- The purpose of the report is to identify the benefits of treating patients as day cases.
- In 1985, The Royal College of Surgeons reported that up to 50% of all postoperative patients need not stay in hospital overnight. Since then, more procedures have become suitable for day case management.
- The main benefits of day surgery are:
    - fast throughput
    - easing pressure on acute surgical specialties
    - reduced waiting lists
    - no deterioration in quality of care
    - savings in hospital 'hotel' costs
    - reduced demand for night and weekend staff
    - making more effective use of operating theatres
    - ease of recruitment and retention of nurses.
- If current levels of day cases were doubled to 30%, £124 million could be saved, or spent on treating more patients.
- Department of Health statistics show that the number of patients receiving day case treatment has doubled in the last 10 years.
- Expansion of day surgery requires a cultural change, with greater involvement by consultants.
- Such change can only be achieved with careful, sensitive planning and agreement of the professions.
- The following key features are recommended as necessary to develop day surgery:
    - capturing the interest and ownership of the concept by surgeons and anaesthetists
    - securing participation by a wide range of specialties
    - provision of dedicated facilities
    - agreed patient selection protocols
    - efficient clerical services
    - ensuring treatment by suitably qualified surgeons and anaesthetists
    - advice to patients
    - sound management.

Published in 1993 by HMSO on behalf of The NHS Management Executive's Value for Money Unit.

- Other recommendations are:
  - provision of adequate space and facilities
  - facilities for teaching in day surgery
  - the encouragement for regional centres in paediatric day surgery
  - improved data collection.

Just for the Day

Establishes principles and standards for children's day case treatment.

RECOMMENDATIONS

- Day care for children should be expanded.
- Children should not be nursed alongside adults.
- Children should be admitted to a children's day ward which admits medical and surgical patients and ward attenders.
- If children are admitted to an adult day unit, there should be separate facilities or separate sessions.

TWELVE QUALITY STANDARDS

A planned package of care for day case admissions:

1. *The admission is planned in an integrated way to include pre-admission, day of admission, and post-admission care, and to incorporate the concept of a planned transfer of care to primary and/or community services.*
2. *The child and parent are offered preparation both before and during the day of admission.*
3. *Specific written information is provided to ensure that parents understand their responsibilities throughout the episode.*
4. *The child is admitted to an area designated for day care and not mixed with acutely ill inpatients.*
5. *The child is neither admitted nor treated alongside adults.*
6. *The child is cared for by identified staff specifically designated to the day case area.*
7. *Medical, nursing and all other staff are trained for, and skilled in, work with children and their families, in addition to the expertise needed for day case work.*
8. *The organisation and delivery of patient care are planned specifically for day cases, so that every child is likely to be discharged within the day.*
9. *The building, equipment and furnishings comply with safety standards for children.*
10. *The environment is homely and includes areas for play and other activities designed for children and young people.*
11. *Essential documentation, including communication with the primary and/or community services, is completed before each child goes home so that after care and follow-up consultations are not delayed.*
12. *Once care has been transferred to the home, nursing support is provided, at a doctor's request, by nurses trained in the care of sick children.*

Published in January 1991 by Caring for Children in the Health Services. The Twelve Quality Standards are reproduced with permission from Action for Sick Children (National Association for the Welfare of Children in Hospital Ltd).

PRINCIPLES UNDERLYING THE ESTABLISHMENT OF A CHILDREN'S DAY PROGRAMME

Environment
The unit should be designed with a homely feel, with childproof fittings. There should be facilities for parents. A treatment room should be equipped to carry out biopsies, chemotherapy, plaster work, etc. All anaesthetic facilities should be to the standard expected in operating theatres.

Staff
There should be a unit director, a manager and nursing staff skilled in the care of sick children. Medical staff should be specifically assigned to the day case service. There should be play staff, health care assistants and clerical staff.

Organisation of patient care
The children's day unit should be part of the children's department. There should be a systematic approach, covering pre-admission, day of admission and post-admission. Guidelines should be drawn up for parents who enter the theatre suite. Managerial and clinical audit should feature prominently.

Delivery of patient care
The consultant decides whether to admit a child on a day basis. A pre-admission programme should be provided. The parent should be able to be with the child whenever he/she is conscious. The number of painful or frightening procedures conducted while the child is conscious should be minimised. Nursing staff should take responsibility for monitoring that the child is ready for discharge. Anaesthetist and surgeon should see the child before discharge.

PRINCIPLES FOR THE MANAGEMENT OF CHILDREN DURING ANAESTHESIA, SURGERY AND RECOVERY

Environment
The anaesthetic and recovery areas should have enough space to allow a parent to participate, and be decorated so as to attract a child's interest. Children should be separated as much as possible in the recovery area.

Staff
Surgeons and anaesthetists working in paediatric day surgery should have appropriate training. The work should be conducted or supervised by consultants.

Organisation of patient care
There should be close co-operation between operating theatre managers and the children's department. Agreed guidelines should be drawn up to help parents in the operating theatre.

Delivery of patient care
The anaesthetist is responsible for deciding fitness for operation. The parent should be allowed into the anaesthetic room whenever possible, the final decision being with the

anaesthetist. During induction of anaesthesia, safety issues are paramount, and if a parent is present he/she should have been prepared for his/her role by staff. The surgeon should employ appropriate means for simplifying postoperative care and patient comfort. There should be one recovery nurse per patient in the recovery area. Anaesthetist and surgeon should see the patient before discharge. The anaesthetist should have agreed the criteria and delegation for discharge.

A Short Cut to Better Services: Day Surgery in England and Wales

Explores cost and other benefits to day surgery.

SUMMARY

- Many surgical procedures can be carried out on a day case basis.
- Day surgery offers two advantages:
    - a service better suited to patient needs, treating patients sooner
    - lower hospital costs.
- Outcomes are no different.
- In spite of this, day surgery is less common in England and Wales than in other countries, and is unevenly distributed.
- If all District Health Authorities performed day surgery for each of 20 common procedures, 186 000 extra patients could be treated at no extra cost. By offering other suitable procedures, 300 000 extra patients could be treated each year. This is equivalent to 34% of existing waiting lists.
- There are obstacles, however:
    - lack of information to estimate potential
    - lack of specialist facilities
    - inappropriate use of existing facilities
    - poor management and organisation of DSUs
    - clinicians' preferences
    - disincentives for managers.
- Many of these obstacles can be overcome. For the first four, the audit commission recommends:
    - a robust method of assessing performance, recording and monitoring progress
    - measures to improve the use made of day case units.
- Financial and management disincentives should be overcome by the purchaser/ provider split.
- Clinician's attitudes are changing gradually.

Published by HMSO on behalf of The Audit Commission.

Report of the Working Party on Guidelines for Day Case Surgery

Recommendations on all aspects of day surgery, including lists of suitable operations.

There has been a growth in the number of day surgery cases treated, but the practice is not yet universally adopted. It is now considered the best option for 50% of all elective surgery, and is popular with patients. There are economic benefits to treatment with day surgery, though financial assessment based on average cost is misleading, and calculations should be based on marginal or opportunity costs.

High standards are required, and trainees should be closely supervised by staff experienced in day surgery.

DEFINITIONS

Surgical day case
A patient admitted for investigations or operation on a planned non-resident basis, and who nonetheless requires facilities for recovery. The definition excludes minor procedures carried out in Accident and Emergency (A&E) or out-patients.

The provision of day surgery is useful for those operations which require a short general anaesthetic and have low morbidity. It may take three forms:

1. Day surgery unit: self-contained, with admission suite, theatre and recovery. This is the ideal.
2. Day surgery ward: for admission of day case patients who are operated on in main theatres on a day case list. This is less desirable.
3. General ward: not recommended. The two main advantages of the day surgery ward, that it is closed out of hours and never blocked with emergency patients, are lost with this arrangement.

Day unit beds may be used for patients undergoing radiological procedures, chronic pain treatment and others.

ACCOMMODATION AND FACILITIES

A ward of 20 beds is the norm, with a range of 10–30. Twelve cases per theatre day is a safe calculation, more if many cases are under local anaesthesia. A 20-bed ward requires two theatres. It is sensible for the last cases in the afternoon to be carried out under local anaesthesia.

Published in March 1992 by The Royal College of Surgeons of England Commission on the Provision of Surgical Services.

Throughput of 1.5 patients per bed day for 240 days per year is possible. If occupancy is no more than 80%, such a unit could treat more than 5750 patients per year.

Location
The ideal is a self-contained unit, ground floor position, with good signposting and an adjacent car park. Proximity to in-patient wards is not essential.

Specifications
Anaesthetic rooms, theatres and recovery areas should be built to the same specification as the in-patient equivalent.

The day ward is best designed on an open plan. A mix of beds and trolleys is desirable. Many procedures may be carried out on trolleys. Minimal bed-head facilities are required. There should be a reception area and an office close by. Other areas, including staff changing rooms, kitchen, equipment store, clean/dirty utility, staff rest room, etc., should be provided on site.

PATIENT SELECTION

- Housing conditions must be satisfactory. If in doubt, confirmation should be sought from the GP or heath visitor. The patient should live no more than 1 hour's drive from the hospital, and have a telephone.
- All patients should be accompanied home, and should not drive. Public transport is not acceptable. Patients should be advised not to operate machinery or cook for 24 hours, or more in some cases. Patients should not drive for at least 48 hours.
- Suitability for day surgery should be assessed at the out-patient consultation, and consent, operation date and investigations arranged then.
- Patients for general anaesthesia should be ASA I or II (ASA I–V = American Society of Anaesthesiologists grading of fitness for anaesthesia). Elderly patients requiring urology procedures who are ASA III or IV may be successfully treated. Gross obesity [body mass index (BMI) >30] is a contraindication.

PREOPERATIVE ROUTINE

The patient should arrive in good time; staggered arrival times are ideal. The anaesthetist sees the patient then. Premedication is usually avoided.

ANAESTHESIA AND POST-ANAESTHETIC RECOVERY

Day surgery requires the highest anaesthetic standards.

The three stages of recovery are:

1. Recovery of vital reflexes such that the patient can be left unattended.
2. Sufficient return of physical and mental functions to return home.
3. Complete psychomotor recovery, enabling driving and use of machinery.

Surgery inevitably interacts with recovery from anaesthesia.

POSTOPERATIVE CARE

- Control of pain is important, using local/regional block, or analgesics by the oral, sublingual or rectal route. Antiemetics may be indicated, but emesis is usually a reflection of postural hypotension and may be relieved on lying down.
- Wounds are best closed with an absorbable subcuticular suture.
- The responsibility for assessment of fitness for discharge rests with the medical staff, but may be delegated to the sister in charge of the ward. The incidence of patients requiring admission overnight should be less than 2–3%.
- The patient and accompanying person should be reminded of the constraints on activity following an anaesthetic. The 24-hour period of restriction will need to be extended to 48 hours when sedatives or opioids are given in conjunction with general, regional or local anaesthesia.
- When sedative or opioid drugs are administered intravenously, even in the absence of general or local anaesthesia, the patient should be observed for a minimum of 1 hour from the last dose.
- When local or regional anaesthesia is given, patients should be warned about the possibility of injury due to loss of sensation.

MANAGEMENT, AUDIT, QUALITY CONTROL

- Each unit should have a clearly stated policy document.
- A clinician should be appointed as director.
- Day-to-day running should be supervised by a nurse manager.
- Accurate information on the activity of the unit should be collected, ideally with the aid of computers. This facilitates audit and quality control.

DAY SURGERY FOR CHILDREN

- Day surgery is highly appropriate for children, but needs careful planning.
- Children should be separated from adult patients, either in a separate day unit or in a general unit reserved for children on one day.
- Skilled anaesthetists and children's nurses should be available.

(A list of appropriate operations for children is provided.)

THE SELECTION OF ADULT SURGICAL PROCEDURES

1. General surgery: haemostasis must be meticulous, and a wound which requires a drain is not generally suitable for day case management. Fine vacuum drains removed before the patient goes home can be used for some procedures.
2. Orthopaedics: image intensifier and plaster facilities should be available.
3. Urology: the need for a urethral catheter used to preclude day case management, but some units have successfully implemented policies of discharge with catheter. Uncatheterised patients should not be discharged until they have passed urine.
4. Ophthalmology procedures are well suited to day case management.
5. ENT: highly suitable (the list does not include tonsillectomy).

6. Plastic surgery: many procedures are ideally suited to day surgery. Flaps and grafts with fine sutures and specialised dressings may need to be seen in a dressings clinic postoperatively rather than by community services.
7. Gynaecology: highly suitable.
8. Oral and maxillofacial surgery: for those procedures requiring general anaesthesia.
9. Thoracic surgery: certain procedures are appropriate, but the small numbers and urgency of the procedure may make efficient use of the unit difficult.

INTERVENTIONAL RADIOLOGY

Fewer procedures requiring hospital admission are carried out, and the majority are performed without general anaesthesia. Arteriography can now safely be performed as a day case.

PAIN RELIEF CLINICS

Many pain clinic procedures require facilities for assessment, an equipped treatment area with image intensifier, facilities for close observation afterwards and secretarial assistance. A DSU provides all these services.

Anaesthetic Services for Obstetrics: A Plan for the Future

Organisation and training for anaesthetic services in different types of obstetric unit.

SUMMARY OF MAIN RECOMMENDATIONS

Immediate action:

- *A named consultant anaesthetist should be responsible for obstetric anaesthetic services in each unit or district. This responsibility should be recognised by the allocation of NHDs.*
- *In small units with infrequent requests for anaesthesia, immediate consideration should be given to the withdrawal of anaesthetic cover. Selection of mothers to be delivered in smaller units should be improved and more emphasis placed on maternal risk factors.*
- *Mothers should be given information if the range of anaesthetic services available in a unit is restricted. Admission to a unit with a comprehensive service should be offered as an alternative.*
- *Courses to train midwives in assistance for the anaesthetist and in adult resuscitation procedures should be introduced.*

Long-term action:

- *Small obstetric units which offer a substandard level of anaesthetic service should be closed, amalgamated or relocated to within a district general hospital or unit where full services are available. A single unit in each district is strongly recommended.*
- *Exceptionally, if it is essential on geographical grounds to maintain an isolated unit, this should be recognised, and recommended levels of anaesthetic staffing allocated to provide the necessary standard of care.*
- *Substandard levels of service should be identified, documented and brought to the attention of Health Authorities and the public. The possible consequences of a substandard level of service should be emphasised.*

Published in October 1987 by The Association of Anaesthetists of Great Britain and Ireland and reproduced with their permission.

Response to the Second Report of the Health Committee on Maternity Services

Comments from the College on the Health Select Committee report, with particular reference to delivery at home or in GP/midwife units.

- The College of Anaesthetists was not invited to present oral evidence to the Select Committee.
- Wider opportunities for choice by mothers is applauded. There is no evidence to prove or disprove the safety of home delivery.
- The Dutch experience is widely quoted, but many important differences exist between this country and Holland. Concerns have been expressed about the safety of home birth in Holland.
- Eighty seven percent of women require pain relief, and home delivery reduces the options available for analgesia.
- Neither small maternity units nor home births can provide the same expertise in neonatal resuscitation as the larger unit. The absence of blood transfusion facilities increases risk, especially in remote areas.
- The report advocates that a second pair of hands be available in case both mother and baby require resuscitation, but does not state where this second pair of hands would come from or how they would be trained. The staffing implications of providing such a basic level of care is enormous, and the outcome is unlikely to be as satisfactory as when occurring in hospital.
- Despite assertions to the contrary by The Royal College of Midwives (RCM), there is no evidence that midwives can deal with all the problems of pregnancy or childbirth, or have the necessary knowledge to refer appropriately.
- Evidence from The Royal College of Obstetricians and Gynaecologists seems not to have been given as much weight in the report as that from other bodies.
- The report places considerable weight on claims by the RCM concerning obstetric intervention, that are unsupported by objective evidence.
- The report suggests that long-term health problems follow childbirth, but no conclusive evidence exists that more home births would reduce this.
- The section on regionalisation of care fails to mention the requirement for high dependency and intensive care facilities.
- Increasing home deliveries would increase the need for flying squads, which would denude the hospital of staff, with risk to other mothers.
- Given that 54% of women initially booked for delivery in midwife/GP units that are part of a specialist unit are transferred to the specialist unit antenatally or during labour, it is unwise to increase booking into geographically separated midwife/GP units.
- The report stresses the need for adequate senior obstetric cover on the labour ward. The College wishes to emphasise the need for adequate senior anaesthetic cover also.

Published in 1992 by The Royal College of Anaesthetists.

- 'Domino' style deliveries would seem to offer the best of both worlds.
- The College would welcome testing the report's recommendations, but only under controlled circumstances in hospital.
- The Health Committee have paid great attention to mothers' desires especially for lower levels of intervention; it is essential that those wishing for greater safety and analgesia are also provided for. The College believes that every mother should have the right to the pain relief she wants, including epidural block.

Anaesthetists and Non-acute Pain Management

Demand, provision, training and audit for non-acute pain management services.

SUMMARY

1. *Many patients might benefit from pain management services.*
2. *There are wide variations in the organisation of pain management services and the availability of assistance.*
3. *It is likely that the number of referrals to pain management units will rise.*
4. *There are no reliable data about pain clinic activity available nationally.*
5. *There are Health Districts that do not provide pain management services.*
6. *Consultant posts with an interest in the management of non-acute pain have been and remain unfilled.*
7. *The lack of suitably trained applicants may be because of insufficient facilities for training, or lack of opportunity to train in pain management.*
8. *There is insufficient teaching about pain and pain management at undergraduate level.*
9. *Pain treatment and pain management services should be available to all who need them.*
10. *National collection of data about activity in pain management units will ensure adequate provision of facilities and budget.*
11. *It is recommended that each medical school curriculum should include structured training in pain management.*
12. *This training should be integrated with other teaching programmes such as palliative care and symptom control.*
13. *It is recommended that anaesthetic trainees at all levels should have adequate experience in pain relief.*
14. *It is recommended that the extent of such training should be defined clearly and commence in the first year of training.*
15. *It is recommended that those participating in Higher Specialist training in anaesthesia should experience a minimum of one month whole time or its sessional equivalent in recognised training in the management of non-acute pain.*
16. *It is recommended that this be increased to three months as improved facilities for training become available.*
17. *It is recommended that those intending to take up a post in anaesthesia and pain management should undergo an additional three month's recognised training.*
18. *It is recommended that full-time post-accreditation posts in pain management be established.*

Published in June 1993 by The Association of Anaesthetists of Great Britain and Ireland, the Royal College of Anaesthetists and the Pain Society and reproduced with permission from The Association of Anaesthetists of Great Britain and Ireland.

Intensive Care Services: Provision for the Future

This report was the product of a national questionnaire survey of 214 intensive care units carried out by the Association.

SUMMARY OF RECOMMENDATIONS

- *Accurate records should be kept. They are essential in the evaluation of intensive care.*
- *A nurse/patient ratio of 1:1 is necessary throughout the 24 hour period.*
- *General intensive care units should have not less than four beds and admit not less than 200 patients per year.*
- *One general intensive care unit should be provided in each Health District. Where the work-load of a district unit is less than that recommended, intensive care services should be provided at a supradistrict level.*
- *Where a hospital has no intensive care unit, patients should be stabilised clinically and then transferred. The process of transfer should be the responsibility of the recipient unit.*
- *An allocation of not less than 15 notional half days (NHDs) per week is required for the size of unit recommended. In 85% of units the work is done by anaesthetists. A majority of these NHDs should therefore be allocated to Departments of Anaesthesia.*
- *Each unit should have a named consultant in administrative charge.*

Published in August 1988 by The Association of Anaesthetists of Great Britain and Ireland and reproduced with their permission.

A Study of Provision of Intensive care in England, 1993: Revised Report of Department of Health

> The result of a survey of patients refused admission to ICU.

EXECUTIVE SUMMARY

- The study has shown that:
    - intensive care provision is unequal between regions
    - reported refusal rates are very variable and depend on bed supply and other factors
    - appropriately referred patients refused admission to a first-choice Intensive Care Unit (ICU) are not much more likely to die than appropriately admitted patients.
- The number of refused requests for admission, like other indices of unmet need, is inadequate as a determinant of bed supply.
- The numbers of admissions were strongly related to supply of facilities (including beds) and this must indicate, in the absence of large differences in unambiguous medical need, that different thresholds for admission criteria to ICUs must exist.
- Considerable numbers of patients were denied the possibility of intensive care because the units were full.
- The study looked at 168 patients refused admission to a study ICU: four were already in an ICU, 34 were admitted to a second-choice ICU, 27 had their admission deferred and 103 were not admitted.
- The study could not show large differences in mortality between refusals and admissions in the six ICUs studied (although possible flaws are suggested to account for this).
- Sixty five percent of admissions designated as inappropriate could have been more appropriately admitted to a High Dependency Unit (HDU).
- There may indeed be a requirement for more high dependency beds. Only 34 of the acute hospitals in England with an ICU had an HDU.
- The costs of supporting patients on HDU is less than on ICU (£600 vs. £1500).
- Supplying intensive care beds on the basis of number of refusals is not a viable option.
- The solution to the problem of intensive care provision can only be reached with outcome studies in well-defined groups of patients.

Published in January 1994 by the Health Promotion Sciences Unit, Department of Public Health & Policy, London School of Hygiene and Tropical Medicine.

Report of the Working Group on Guidelines on Admission to and Discharge from Intensive Care and High Dependency Units

Recommendations on audit, organisation and contracting for intensive care services. Guidelines for admission and discharge published separately.

RECOMMENDATIONS

Guidelines
The Working Group has produced guidelines for issue to intensive care staff as well as for other staff in hospitals who are involved in referring patients to intensive care or high dependency care and for the attention of purchasers of intensive care. It is recommended that these guidelines are issued to the NHS as soon as possible.

Specialty status
The Working Group hopes that the Royal Colleges will address the designation of intensive care as a specialty as soon as possible in view of the potential service benefits including improved quality of care.

Data requirements
The Working Group recommends that there should be routine collection of data as Finished Consultant Episodes or as Intensive Care Episodes on patients given intensive and high dependency care which should form part of the Contract Minimum Data Set. The group welcomes the initial progress made towards this initiative and recommends that these changes should be introduced on 1 April 1997.

The Working Group recommends that Healthcare Resource Groups should be developed as a more accurate way of allocating costs in intensive care.

The Working Group recommends that participation in collaborative clinical audit by ICUs is encouraged as a way of developing a consensus on case-mix measurement for audit and research purposes.

Contracting
The Working Group recommends that NHS purchasers should be involved in decisions about the allocation of resources to intensive care and high dependency care and in contracting for these services.

The Royal College of Anaesthetists and the Intensive Care Society have produced guidelines for purchasers of anaesthetic services including intensive care. The Working Group recommends this guidance and recommends that, once more detailed information is available on intensive

Published in March 1996 by the Department of Health and reproduced with their permission.

care and high dependency care, the NHS Executive should consider the need for further guidelines on contracting for these services to facilitate the complete integration of intensive care and high dependency care into the NHS internal market.

Consultant sessional allocation

The Working Group recommends that consultant sessional allocation to intensive care should be reviewed and, where appropriate, increased to ensure that decisions on admissions, discharges and transfers are made by experienced, senior clinicians.

Further work

- Outcome of intensive care and high dependency care.

  The Working Group recommends that further research should be carried out to evaluate the outcome of intensive care and high dependency care.

- Nursing
  - In order for useful comparisons to be made with other European countries and the US (and inform discussion about the relevance of recommendations from US research studies and policy recommendations), it is recommended that further evidence should be made available from the other countries regarding:
    - case-mix; there is preliminary evidence from the EURICUS-I study to suggest that the UK intensive care population is more severely ill than in other European countries;
    - the nature of nursing work;
    - the roles of members of the multidisciplinary team (medical, nursing and support staff).
  - The Working Group recommends that a study should be undertaken to examine dependency and the association between dependency and resource usage, in particular nursing resources.
- Bed state register
  - The Working Group recommends that an options appraisal should be carried out to compare the costs and benefits of a computerised with a manual bed state register.

Guidelines on Admission to and Discharge from Intensive Care and High Dependency Units

Advice on efficient use of high dependency and intensive care resources.

INTRODUCTION

- There is a lack of consensus on the definition of intensive care/high dependency beds, and on the best use of these facilities.
- There may be scope for improving efficiency by excluding patients who are not ill enough or too ill.
- Local agreed protocols should be devised based on these guidelines.
- These guidelines define categories of care rather than geographical areas of the hospital.

DEFINITIONS

- These definitions apply mainly to general medical and surgical patients, and also to cardiac and neurosurgical intensive care. Renal units, coronary care, paediatric and neonatal intensive care are outside the scope of these guidelines.
- Intensive care is *"a service for patients with potentially recoverable conditions who can benefit from more detailed observation and invasive treatment than can safely be provided in general wards or high dependency areas"*.
- High dependency care provides a level of care intermediate between that on a general ward and intensive care. It monitors and supports patients with or likely to develop, acute single organ failure. It should not manage multiorgan failure or mechanical ventilation.
- High dependency care provided in a unit adjacent to intensive care provides better medical care than an isolated unit without specialist cover from the intensive care team.

(Detailed descriptions of the characteristics of intensive care and high dependency care are provided.)

GUIDELINES FOR ADMISSION TO INTENSIVE CARE

Referral
- Where possible, referral should be made by a consultant, and the patient should ideally be seen by the intensive care consultant before admission.
- Delegation to trainee doctors should be made only where clear guidelines and appropriate training are provided.

Published in March 1996 by the Department of Health.

Reversibility of illness

- The degree of benefit from intensive care admission depends on whether the patient has a reversible illness. This may be difficult to assess in some cases, but patients should not be offered treatment inappropriately.
- Decisions should be made jointly by patient, family, intensive care team and referring team.
- Patients with persistent vegetative state should not be admitted to intensive care, nor should competent patients who refuse such care.
- The practice of interventional ventilation (therapy provided not for the patient's benefit but for the purposes of organ donation) is not permitted.

Co-morbidity

Pre-existing chronic organ system impairment must be taken into account when considering the potential benefits of intensive care.

Patients' advanced statements

A patient's written or stated preference against intensive care should be taken into account.

Advanced respiratory support

The decision as to whether advanced respiratory support is required rests with the intensive care doctor.

Other acute organ support

Intensive care should be provided for those who, although not needing ventilatory support, require support for two or more other organ systems.

Dependency

The level of dependency is an important factor in determining the appropriateness of intensive care.

Objective criteria to determine benefit of admission to intensive care

- The outcome measure used to audit intensive care is hospital mortality. A number of risk adjustment methods have been developed for intensive care, for example APACHE, SAPS and MPM.
- The evidence to support the use of risk adjustment measures to decide whether to admit an individual patient is weak. They may, however, assist in decision making, and are a useful audit and research tool.

GUIDELINES ON ADMISSION TO HIGH DEPENDENCY CARE

- The appropriateness of intensive care admission depends on what other facilities are available.
- Establishing an intermediate level of care can reduce ward mortality rates by 25% and cardiac arrests by 39%.
- Patients requiring support of one organ system (excluding advanced respiratory support) should receive high dependency care.

- High dependency care may be warranted for the patient who is not undergoing medical intervention, but needs to be closely monitored.

GUIDELINES ON DISCHARGE FROM INTENSIVE CARE AND HIGH DEPENDENCY CARE

- A patient may be discharged from intensive care when the condition requiring referral has been reversed, or when the intensive care consultant considers that the patient will no longer benefit from the treatment available.
- Many patients remain on intensive care longer than necessary in the absence of an HDU.
- Hospital mortality following intensive care is reported at 6–16%, but the risk of death may be reduced if high dependency facilities are available.

Treatment limitation/withdrawal

- Assessment of continuing appropriateness of intensive care should be made at least daily.
- A decision to limit further treatment should be made after discussion with the referring team, and should have the full acceptance and understanding of the patient and relatives.
- When treatment is limited, the aims if intensive care should change so that the patient is made comfortable. Moving the patient from the unit may cause difficulty for family and staff.

Organ donation

Organ donors should stay on ICU until the organs are retrieved. The resource implications of this are significant.

CONSULTANT SESSIONAL ALLOCATION

- The Intensive Care Society recommends that for units of up to 10 beds, there should be a minimum of 15 consultant sessions shared between three or four individuals.
- Many ICUs do not meet this allocation.

NURSE STAFFING

- Bed closures are frequently due to lack of trained nursing staff.
- A nurse:patient ratio of 1:1 is considered essential.
- The nurse:patient ratio adopted in the UK is generally higher than in other European countries.

TRANSFERS BETWEEN ICUs

- Transfer of patients between ICUs is an integral part of the intensive care service.
- Fluctuations in the demand for intensive care and high dependency beds will inevitably lead to occasions when patients need to be transferred.
- Transfers should be kept to a minimum, as they are potentially dangerous, but it is now possible to move the patient without his/her condition deteriorating.

- To achieve safe transfer, the aim should be to move the intensive care environment with the patient.
- It may be more appropriate to transfer a stabler, less sick ICU patient, rather than the one requiring admission, subject to discussions with patient, relatives and consultant(s) responsible for his/her care.

ARRANGING THE TRANSFER

- Transfer should involve formal referral of care from consultant to consultant.
- The standards of monitoring should be the same as within the ICU. Experienced staff should accompany the patient.

Preparation
The patient must be resuscitated adequately prior to transfer.

Monitoring
- The patient requires: electrocardiography (ECG), pulse oximetry, blood pressure measurement (preferably with an arterial line), capnography, two or more intravenous lines, urinary catheter, body temperature monitoring and airway pressure monitoring.
- If a pulmonary artery catheter is *in situ* then continuous monitoring of the waveform is required.
- Recording the monitoring during transfer is essential.

Equipment
- Basic equipment of a mobile ICU is a vehicle and purpose-built trolley.
- Hand ventilation is unsatisfactory.
- Equipment required includes: provision for artificial ventilation with PEEP, equipment and drugs for airway management, capnograph, portable syringe drivers, suction, intra-arterial pressure monitoring equipment, battery-powered pulse oximeter, Wrights spirometer or similar, HME, defibrillator, warming blanket.
- Accompanying staff must be familiar with all aspects of care of the critically ill.

Sedation and Anaesthesia in Radiology: Recommendations of the Joint Working Party of The Royal College of Radiologists and The Royal College of Anaesthetists

Issues relating to sedation, anaesthesia and resuscitation in radiology departments, conducted with or without the presence of an anaesthetist.

DEFINITIONS

Sedation is defined as 'a technique in which the use of a drug or drugs produces a state of depression of the central nervous system enabling treatment to be carried out but during which verbal contact with the patient is maintained throughout the period of sedation. The drugs and techniques used should carry a margin of safety wide enough to render unintended loss of consciousness unlikely'.

Anaesthesia is defined as 'any technique in which a drug or combination of drugs produces loss of consciousness, as defined by a failure to respond to verbal command'.

PATIENT SELECTION

Patients should undergo medical screening. The responsibility for screening tests rests with the radiologist. Checklists may be useful.

SEDATION IN RADIOLOGY DEPARTMENTS

Sedation should be carried out under the responsibility of a named consultant radiologist. A trained assistant should be present to monitor the patient. Agreed guidelines should exist on drugs and maximum doses. Anaesthetic assistance should be rapidly available when required. For children, the presence of a parent should be encouraged.

ANAESTHESIA IN RADIOLOGY DEPARTMENTS

This should be conducted by an anaesthetist, and not on the same day as a failed procedure under sedation. Skilled anaesthetic assistance should be available.

RECOVERY

Adequate recovery facilities should be available.

Published in July 1992 by The Royal College of Anaesthetists.

EQUIPMENT

Wherever sedation or anaesthesia is given in radiology departments, the area should be equipped for resuscitation. Equipment should include oxygen, suction, drugs, stethoscope, non-invasive blood pressure, pulse oximeter, ECG, defibrillator, and the usual anaesthetic drugs, equipment and monitoring. A tipping trolley should be available. Children's equipment and drug dosage charts should be available.

THE ROLE OF THE ANAESTHETIST IN THE RADIOLOGY DEPARTMENT

Anaesthetists are likely to be involved in the radiology department for patient assessment, anaesthesia, radiology for critically ill patients and emergencies occurring in the department.

A designated anaesthetist should take responsibility for anaesthetic matters in the radiology department, dealing with guidelines for sedation, definition of training and supervision, patient selection criteria, monitoring, drug information, data recording and audit.

He/she should also ensure provision of resuscitation equipment and drugs, provide advice on drugs and room design, and advise on training in matters of sedation and anaesthesia.

RESUSCITATION

All staff should be familiar with resuscitation methods, and undergo periodic reassessment and retraining. Radiologists should be trained in the use of sedative drugs, and all nurses and radiographers should be trained in monitoring of sedated patients and the detection of adverse reactions.

Report of the Joint Working Party on Anaesthesia in Ophthalmic Surgery

Clinical guidelines relating to eye surgery performed under local anaesthesia.

- Major eye surgery is increasingly performed under local anaesthesia. Concern was expressed about such operations being performed in the absence of an anaesthetist. Complications may occur during such procedures, and the surgeon cannot monitor the patient adequately while concentrating on the surgery.
- Preoperative evaluation is important whether general anaesthesia or local anaesthesia is used. Preoperative investigations should be ordered, regardless of anaesthetic technique, as follows:
  - ECG: for patients over 60 and those with cardiovascular disease.
  - Chest X-ray: for patients with chronic lung disease, or any suggestion of tuberculosis or malignancy.
  - Urea and electrolytes: on patients over 60, those with renal disease, and those on cardiac, renal or steroid drugs.
  - Blood sugar: for diabetics and patients on steroids.
  - Haemoglobin: all women, men over 60, and those with signs of anaemia.
- Monitoring for operations under local anaesthesia should include verbal contact, pulse oximetry, ECG and blood pressure measurement. Intravenous access should always be obtained.
- A trained nurse or operating department assistant (ODA) could perform the task of monitoring the patient, but could not take remedial action when necessary.
- The Working Party agreed, therefore, that an anaesthetist should be present to monitor the patient's condition throughout the operation, and provide resuscitation if necessary.
- It was also suggested that the anaesthetist should also be responsible for advising on the appropriateness of local or general anaesthesia, prescribing sedation where necessary, giving the local block and providing intravenous access, and supervising the postoperative recovery.
- Minor procedures requiring infiltration anaesthesia do not need the presence of an anaesthetist.

LOCAL ANAESTHESIA FOR CATARACT SURGERY – BACKGROUND INFORMATION

Introduction
Fifty percent of cataract surgery currently is carried out under local anaesthesia. Complications can occur, especially when the technique is reserved for the least fit or is combined with sedation.

Published in March 1993 by The Association of Anaesthetists of Great Britain and Ireland and The College of Ophthalmologists.

Life-threatening complications have occurred in 1:750 anaesthetics administered, and serious complications in 1:360. With 60 000 local anaesthesia cataract operations per year, this means 80 life-threatening complications and 170 serious complications may be anticipated.

Forms of local anaesthesia
1. Retrobulbar block: can cause globe perforation, and direct injection into the optic nerve sheath.
2. Peribulbar block: is said to be safer, but equally effective. It is not as effective at producing akinesia.
3. Topical anaesthesia, combined with phacoemulsification, is being evaluated.

Sedation
Sedation is defined as the use of a drug or drugs which produce a state of depression of the central nervous system (CNS) enabling treatment to be carried out, but during which verbal contact is maintained with the patient throughout. The drugs and techniques used should carry a margin of safety wide enough to render unintended unconsciousness unlikely.

Specific disorders commonly occurring in patients for cataract surgery
Hypertensive patients should have blood pressure controlled before surgery, to reduce the chance of myocardial ischaemia, up 70% of which is silent.

Valvular heart disease needs careful assessment. Antibiotic prophylaxis is not necessary.

Patients on anticoagulant therapy should have an International Normalised Ratio (INR) no greater than 2.0.

Patients with chronic obstructive airways disease (COAD) may need control of factors causing coughing. Those with a raised arterial P_aCO_2 on air are at risk of respiratory depression from high inspired oxygen concentrations. A more open system of draping may be necessary.

Diabetics: blood glucose should be 5–10 mmol/l, ideally on the normal regimen. Preparation as for general anaesthesia is an alternative.

Patients on steroids may require additional doses.

Adverse incident reports
The Working Party report is appended by an adverse incident report form, which can be filled in and returned to the College of Ophthalmologists.

Surgery and General Anaesthesia in General Practitioner Premises

Issues of provision of service, quality, supplies and professional matters relating to surgery performed in general practitioner premises.

GPs are being encouraged to undertake surgical procedures within their practice premises, some requiring general anaesthesia or sedation.

Although the majority of procedures will be minor operations under local anaesthesia, there may be a wish in some practices to perform more complex surgery.

Those providing the service must be sufficiently well trained and experienced.

Surgery in children requiring general anaesthesia should not be carried out in general practice premises.

FACILITIES

Services should be consultant based, carried out by holders of the Certificate of Completion of Specialist Training (CCST) or equivalent, who are trained in resuscitation.

Skilled, dedicated anaesthetic assistance, nursing staff and recovery staff should be available.

There should be facilities for preoperative assessment, and investigations. Patient identification and discharge should be as for hospital practice. There should be guidelines for the management of rare complications, mechanisms to allow the surgeon and anaesthetists to be contacted, and facilities for transfer in the event of serious complications.

SPECIALIST SERVICES

Drugs, anaesthetic equipment, monitoring and resuscitation facilities should be equivalent to those in hospital.

Surgical services must conform with the Royal College of Surgeons Working Party report on day case surgery (see page 11).

STERILISATION SERVICES

Sterile supplies will either be 'bought in' or produced at the surgery. Relevant standards must be maintained in either case.

Published in March 1995 by The Association of Anaesthetists of Great Britain and Ireland.

TECHNICAL SERVICES

Anaesthetic resuscitation and monitoring equipment needs to be serviced and staff trained in its maintenance. The premises should receive the appropriate Hazard Warning Notices.

Cylinders of medical gases should be stored in accordance with the regulations in Health Technical Memorandum (HTM) 2022 *Medical gas pipeline systems* (NHS Estates 1994).

Volatile agents must be stored and transferred appropriately.

Extraction of waste gases must also conform to HTM 2022.

QUALITY, FINANCIAL AND CONTRACTUAL ARRANGEMENTS

The quality of patient care must not be compromised.

Trusts may not permit consultants to undertake such work.

Income from such work will be deemed as private practice and subject to the 10% limit for full time consultants. The work will not be covered by NHS indemnity.

General Anaesthesia, Sedation and Resuscitation in Dentistry. Report of an Expert Working Party ('The Poswillo Report')

Staffing, training, equipment and clinical guidelines for anaesthesia, sedation and resuscitation in dental practices.

DEFINITIONS

Simple dental sedation is defined as "*a carefully controlled technique in which a single intravenous drug, or a combination of oxygen and nitrous oxide, is used to reinforce hypnotic suggestion and reassurance in a way which allows dental treatment to be performed with minimal physiological and psychological stress, but which allows verbal contact with the patient to maintained at all times. The technique must carry a margin of safety wide enough to render unintended loss of consciousness unlikely*". Anything else is considered as dental general anaesthesia.

GENERAL ANAESTHESIA

1. The use of general anaesthesia should be avoided if at all possible.
2. The same general standards of personnel, premises and equipment should apply wherever general anaesthesia is administered.
3. Dental anaesthesia must be regarded as a postgraduate subject.
4. All anaesthesia should be administered by accredited anaesthetists. Anaesthetic training should include experience in dental anaesthesia.
5. The provision of consultant dental anaesthetic sessions should be reviewed to ensure local needs are met.
6. Doctors and dentists with knowledge, experience and competence sufficient to satisfy the College of Anaesthetists and the faculty of Dental Surgery should be under no detriment. The no detriment arrangements must have been implemented within 2 years of this report.
7. The administration of general anaesthesia in dental surgeries equipped to the recommended standard of monitoring shall continue.
8. ECG, pulse oximeter and non-invasive blood pressure measurement are essential for general anaesthesia. A capnograph should be used with 'tracheal anaesthesia' [note from author: assumed to mean general anaesthesia involving tracheal intubation]. A defibrillator must be available.
9. Equipment conforming to recognised standards should be installed and regularly serviced. General anaesthesia surgeries should be inspected and registered.
10. Intravenous agents should be administered via an indwelling needle or cannula which should not be removed until the patient has fully recovered.
11. Appropriate training should be provided for those assisting the anaesthetists and dentist.

Published in March 1990 by The Standing Dental Advisory Committee.

12. There should be adequate facilities for recovery. The recovering patient should never be left unattended.
13. Contemporaneous records of all treatments should be kept. Written consent should be obtained before general anaesthesia. Consideration should be given to developing a national general anaesthetic/sedation consent form for general dental practitioners.
14. Patients should be provided with comprehensive pre- and post-treatment instructions and advice.

SEDATION

1. Sedation should be used in preference to general anaesthesia wherever possible.
2. For sedation by inhalation, the minimum oxygen concentration should be fixed at 30%.
3. A British standard for relative analgesia machines should be developed.
4. Flumazenil should be reserved for emergency use.
5. Intravenous sedation should be limited to the use of one drug with a single titrated dose and an end point remote from anaesthesia.
6. Intravenous sedation should be approached with caution in children.
7. Practical training in sedation for dentistry should be provided by dentists.
8. More emphasis should be given to undergraduate education in sedation. Undergraduates should be proficient in venepuncture. They should have had experience in administering inhalational sedation in at least 10 cases, and intravenous sedation in at least five cases.
9. Interested dentists should complete a recognised course in sedation within 2 years of qualification.
10. Dentists should be aware of the significance of pulse oximetry readings.
11. All patients should give written consent to treatment, and be given written pre- and postoperative instructions. Patients treated with sedation should be accompanied by a responsible person.

RESUSCITATION

- Every member of the dental team should be trained in resuscitation, and have their proficiency tested and certified.
- Resuscitation procedures should be practised regularly.
- Medical history should be obtained before any treatment.
- Every practice should have a copy of 'ABC of Resuscitation', and be familiar with its contents.
- Dentists must be proficient in the use of airway adjuncts.
- Dental students should be taught basic life support very early in the course.
- All dental anaesthetists should have advanced life support skills.
- Dental surgeries should be equipped to enable resuscitation to be performed. The following drugs should be available:
  - First line resuscitation drugs:
    oxygen, adrenaline, lignocaine, atropine, calcium chloride, sodium bicarbonate, glyceryl trinitrate.

-   Second line drugs:
    aminophylline, salbutamol, chlorpheniramine, 50% dextrose, hydrocortisone, flumazenil, naloxone, midazolam, suxamethonium, dextrose/saline, colloid solution.
    Stocks of drugs should be reviewed regularly.
-   In addition, further appropriate items of resuscitation equipment should be available (these are listed in detail in the original document).

FINANCIAL IMPLICATIONS AND OTHER MATTERS

1. The Department of Health and the profession should consider the financial implications of these recommendations.
2. Sufficient funds should be made available for postgraduate training in general anaesthesia, sedation and resuscitation.
3. An ongoing enquiry into dental general anaesthesia and sedation should be set up.

Joint Response to the SDAC Report on General Anaesthesia, Sedation and Resuscitation in Dentistry

Comments and suggested amendments to the 'Poswillo Report' (see page 33) from The Royal College of Anaesthetists and The Faculty of Dental Surgery.

The College and Faculty warmly welcome and approve the 'Poswillo Report', and comments on it are intended to be constructive. Many recommendations are agreed without reservation.

DEFINITIONS

The definitions confuse the technique with the physiological state produced. Modified definitions are suggested. The principle that dental sedation should be an adjuvant to local anaesthesia is a major omission.

It is recommended that 'Principal Recommendations (Definitions)' should read:

1. *Sedation is a state of reduced consciousness in which verbal contact with the patient is maintained throughout.*
2. *The aim of sedation is to allow dental treatment to be performed, including the use of local anaesthesia when indicated, with minimal stress and pain.*
3. *Sedation has limitations and failures. There are circumstances where therefore general anaesthesia will be required. On the other hand, effective use of nerve blocks will reduce the need for either sedation or general anaesthesia.*
4. *Sedation may be reinforced by the use of reassurance and hypnotic suggestion as well as pharmacological agents.*
5. *Simple sedation is defined as that produced by a combination of oxygen (minimum 30%) and restricted nitrous oxide (30%) or a single titrated intravenous drug.*
6. *It is recognised that sedation may also be achieved by the use of mixtures of drugs. If verbal contact is maintained this is still true sedation. However, the use of such mixtures is complex and inherently less controllable. Their use in dentistry should be subject to specific restrictions as recommended in the Report.*
7. *Sedation techniques should only be used by those whose training and experience ensures a margin of safety wide enough to render unintended loss of verbal contact or unconsciousness unlikely.*
8. *General anaesthesia is a condition of controlled loss of consciousness such that verbal contact is lost. This complex and potentially dangerous condition should always be administered by those adequately trained supported by appropriate facilities.*

Published by The Faculty of Dental Surgery and The Royal College of Anaesthetists and reproduced with their permission.

GENERAL ANAESTHESIA

A different emphasis is recommended, together with additions. Reference is made to the Spence Report (1979). Anaesthesia, while only practised after postgraduate training, is a subject which must be part of the undergraduate course.

Suggested modifications to 'Principal Recommendations (General anaesthesia)':

- The basic principles of the science and clinical practice of anaesthesia should continue to be taught to all dental and medical undergraduates.
- Unsupervised dental anaesthetics should only be administered by medical or dental practitioners who have undertaken approved postgraduate training.
- The training of consultant anaesthetists should be strengthened with further specific supervised experience in dental anaesthesia.
- It is not suggested that the administration of general anaesthetics in suitable dental surgeries shall cease. Suitable surgeries and equipment are described in the Spence Report, 3.0 to 7.0.
- A pulse oximeter, a non-invasive blood pressure device and an ECG in that order of priority are essential for the non-invasive monitoring of a patient under general anaesthesia.
- A capnograph should be used where 'tracheal anaesthesia' [note from author: assumed to mean general anaesthesia involving tracheal anaesthesia] is practised.
- A defibrillator, equipped with both adult and paediatric paddles, must be available.
- Adequate suction and an operating light including standby equipment should be available.
- The competent authority, responsible for inspecting and registering general anaesthetic surgeries, should be identified.
- It should be stated that general anaesthesia will remain unavoidable for many patients, for example handicapped patients, where local anaesthesia has failed or is contraindicated, for multiple extractions, (especially in children), and for highly nervous patients.
- There is no place for the single handed operator/anaesthetist.
- The supine position is essential for patients undergoing general anaesthesia, and helpful for sedation.

SEDATION

Modifications to 'Principal Recommendations (Sedation)':

- Where possible, simple sedation should be used in preference to general anaesthesia.
- For simple sedation, an inhalation machine should be used which delivers a concentration of not less than 30% oxygen and a maximum of 30% nitrous oxide by volume. The equipment should ensure that in the event of failure there is free ingress of air and that the nitrous oxide supply is automatically cut off.
- Flumazenil should be reserved for emergency use and not used routinely to speed recovery.
- Simple sedation by the intravenous route shall be limited to the use of one drug. One single dose titrated to an end point remote from anaesthesia should be used.
- Practical training in simple sedation for dentistry may be provided by dentists.

- Undergraduate or postgraduate courses in sedation should include an update in the relevant basic sciences. All dentists practising sedation should take refresher courses regularly.
- Undergraduates should be instructed in patient management with intravenous sedation.
- Resources should be provided to allow Postgraduate Deans to organise courses in simple sedation. This should include and be combined with training in effective local and regional anaesthesia.

RESUSCITATION

The recommendations should discriminate between skills and facilities required to protect the patient from the clinical techniques practised, and those which may be desirable in order to offer a life support service to the public at large.

Second line drugs are not essential to a dental practice unless general anaesthesia is administered.

Dental General Anaesthesia

A report on the provision of general anaesthesia for dentistry.

SUMMARY OF FINDINGS

1. *There has been a reduction of 14% in item 24(a) claims [i.e. those for general anaesthesia] in the General Dental Services (GDS) in the last two years. The change is not consistent throughout England and Wales: the Thames Regions showed an increase in the number of general anaesthetics administered in the GDS.*
2. *The GDS remains the major provider of general anaesthesia for dental treatment. Within the GDS less than 20% of General Dental Practitioners (GDPs) provide facilities for dental treatment under general anaesthesia. The top 1% claimants made 399 or more claims.*
3. *There has been an increase in all regions in the provision of general anaesthesia by the Community Dental Services (CDS) which, nationally matches the decrease in 24(a) claims in the GDS.*
4. *Information on hospital activity for general anaesthesia for dental treatment is poor. There is little evidence to suggest that there has been a move from the GDS to Hospital Dental Services (HDS). The total general anaesthesia provision for routine dental treatment in the HDS is small.*
5. *Community Health Councils (CHCs) and Family Health Service Authorities (FHSAs) have had very few complaints concerning the provision of general anaesthesia for dental treatment.*
6. *Over one-third of dentists receiving referrals for dental treatment under general anaesthesia expressed concern at the poor quality of referral letters.*
7. *45% of GDPs use the service of a consultant anaesthetist when providing dental general anaesthesia. The anaesthetist provides most of the equipment and anaesthetic drugs. GDPs provide premises, other equipment and staff. Where GDPs are major providers they are largely responsible for providing anaesthetic and monitoring equipment, drugs and auxiliary personnel as well as having financial responsibility for premises and staff.*
8. *In the CDS the majority of anaesthetics are provided by consultant anaesthetists. Equipment, drugs and auxiliary staff are provided by the CDS.*
9. *The average distance travelled for a general anaesthetic in the GDS was 7 miles. In the CDS the mean distance travelled was 6 miles.*
10. *On the GDS waiting times overall were less than 2 weeks. Urgent cases were likely to be seen quickly. In the CDS the average waiting time was 22 days, with some recorded exceptions.*
11. *The CDS treats mainly children, the majority of whom require extraction of carious deciduous teeth. The GDS treats mainly children who require the extraction of deciduous and permanent teeth.*
12. *The 'major providers' in the GDS expect to continue providing a service. They anticipate an increase in the number of referrals that are made to them.*

13. *Despite acknowledging problems with the provision of general anaesthesia in the GDS, over 70% of anaesthetists involved intend to continue the service they provide. They are concerned about the poor levels of training of auxiliary staff.*
14. *The clinical visits together with information from the questionnaires cause concern over shortfalls in standards of patient care and monitoring, safety and resuscitation training for ancillary staff.*
15. *The majority of dental general anaesthetics are given for the routine extraction of teeth and many may not fulfil the published criteria for such an anaesthetic.*
16. *A significant number of general anaesthetics are being given on demand rather than because of clinical need.*
17. *The current fee structure in the GDS is inappropriate for the provision of a general anaesthetic service.*

RECOMMENDATIONS

These recommendations are directed to those we believe have the principal interest in their implementation. Others will be required to ensure their achievement. Positive support for Dental Practice Health preventative initiatives should continue. All should endeavour to encourage the trend towards a reduction in the use of unnecessary general anaesthesia for dentistry.

The professions

Standards should be established for patient care, safety, facilities and training for dentists, anaesthetists and supporting staff, including criteria for appropriate selection of patients for general anaesthesia for dentistry. Achievement should be audited against those standards in all practices and centres where general anaesthesia for dentistry is provided, including arrangements for periodic inspection of facilities.

Improved referral procedures for general anaesthesia for dentistry, acceptable to both the referring dentist and the operative dental and anaesthetic teams, should be established. Standardised informed consent agreements should be developed.

Educational initiatives extending skills in patient management and pain control should be promoted at both undergraduate and postgraduate levels, with the aim of changing attitudes.

Purchasing/commissioning bodies

Commissioners of services should monitor waiting times for dental treatments under general anaesthesia.

Concentration of general anaesthesia for dentistry services in specialist centres should be encouraged by targeting resources on specialist practices or centres, including day care surgery units.

The health departments

Consideration of the method of remuneration for general anaesthesia for dental treatment within the GDS in the light of proposals in the Government Discussion Paper 'Improving NHS Dentistry' should specifically take account of its effect on demand for general anaesthesia for dentistry.

A prospective study of morbidity in all settings, including the development of precise measures of the outcomes of Dental General Anaesthetics, should be commissioned. Comparable data collection from the GDS, CDS and HDS is necessary.

Anaphylactic Reactions Associated with Anaesthesia

This is the first of the Association's two documents on the subject.

SUMMARY

1. *Anaphylactic reactions are rare during anaesthesia; even severe reactions show a prompt and successful response to appropriate treatment in most patients.*
2. *Every anaesthetist should know an 'anaphylaxis drill'.*
3. *Anaesthetists should rehearse a simulated 'anaphylaxis drill' at regular intervals.*
4. *Treatment normally should include adrenaline intravenously at an early stage, particularly in the presence of bronchospasm.*
5. *Any patient who has a suspected anaphylactic reaction associated with anaesthesia should be investigated fully.*
6. *Skin tests are the most readily available and useful test for drug allergy. We recommend the prick test in the investigation of anaphylaxis associated with anaesthesia.*
7. *If it is known that the skin test is positive for a drug, the patient must not receive the drug again.*
8. *Further studies are necessary to show the clinical relevance of the results of RAST investigations.*
9. *All adverse events should be reported to the Committee on Safety of Medicines.*
10. *There is no valid predictor of drug anaphylaxis at present. Claims that any form of screening will predict anaphylaxis are without foundation.*

Published in September 1990 by The Association of Anaesthetists of Great Britain and Ireland and reproduced with their permission.

Suspected Anaphylactic Reactions Associated with Anaesthesia

Incidence, management, investigation and reporting of anaphylactic reactions. Updates 'Anaphylactic Reactions Associated with Anaesthesia' (1990) (see page 41).

- The incidence of these reactions is not known with certainty, but there are estimated to be 175–1000 reactions in the UK per year. Reactions are 3–10 times more common in women, and more common with intravenous injections. In up to 80% of cases there is no history of prior exposure to the precipitating agent. Latex allergy is a relatively common cause of anaphylaxis, especially during abdominal or gynaecological surgery. The reaction typically begins 30–60 minutes into the procedure. Patients allergic to latex may also have food allergies.
- The clinical features of anaphylaxis are cardiovascular collapse (88%), bronchospasm (36%) angio-oedema of face (24%), generalised oedema (7%), rash (13%) erythema (45%), urticaria (8.5%)
- Any suspected reaction should be investigated. The anaesthetist who administered the drugs is responsible for initiating the investigations and giving advice to the patient. Investigations should be conducted in consultation with a clinical immunologist. A list of names and addresses is published by the British Society of Allergy and Clinical Immunology, and is available from the Association of Anaesthetists.
- Ten millilitres of venous blood should be taken for serum tryptase measurement. The serum should be separated, and stored at –20°C until it can be sent to a reference laboratory. Tryptase is found principally in mast cells, and a raised plasma concentration is consistent with generalised mast cell degranulation. Concentrations are maximal at approximately 1 hour after the reaction. Tryptase can be measured post mortem.
- No blood test can confidently identify the causative agent. A full account of events and a detailed history from the patient including known allergies, intercurrent illnesses and previous anaesthetic history should be taken. The Working Party recommends that skin prick tests **when carried out by a person experienced in the technique** offer the best hope of identifying the causative agent. Antibodies to a limited range of anaesthetic agents may be detected by serological tests. Except in the case of suxamethonium, specific radioallergosorbent (RAST) tests have been abandoned.
- All serious reactions should be reported to the Committee on Safety of Medicines, using the yellow card system. The patient and the GP should be informed.
- Screening tests are of no value. The 'test dose' is not an appropriate way of screening for anaphylaxis. Fatal reactions have occurred after very small doses.

Revised edition published in October 1995 by The Association of Anaesthetists of Great Britain and Ireland, and The British Society of Allergy and Clinical Immunology. First edition published in September 1990.

Treatment of anaphylaxis

- **Initial therapy**: stop administration, maintain airway, give 100% oxygen. Lay patient flat with feet elevated. Give adrenaline **either** 0.5–1.0 mg intramuscularly, repeated every 10 minutes where necessary, **or** 50–100 µg intravenously over 1 minute, repeated as required. In a patient with cardiovascular collapse, 0.5–1 mg may be given intravenously. Give intravenous volume expansion with crystalloid or colloid.
- **Secondary therapy**: chlorpheniramine 10–20 mg intravenously, hydrocortisone 100–300 mg intravenously, catecholamine infusions, bicarbonate where acidotic, bronchodilators for persistent bronchospasm. Evaluate airway before extubation.

Checklist for Anaesthetic Machines

These guidelines are universally accepted to be the definitive standard for anaesthetic machine checks.

INTRODUCTION

- Checking the correct functioning of anaesthetic apparatus before use is mandatory. This document updates the procedure recommended in the previous version, published in 1990.
- A major cause of anaesthetic misadventure is use of a machine which has not been adequately checked by an anaesthetist beforehand. Use of checklists and associated procedures should be seen as an integral part of training in anaesthesia.
- This checklist should be applicable to all anaesthetic machines. It should supplement, not supplant, any pre-anaesthetic checking procedures issued by manufacturers.
- The checklist is based, as before, on the obligatory use of an oxygen analyser on every machine.
- It is strongly recommended that a record of the checks be kept.

PROCEDURES

The following checks should be carried out at the beginning of each operating theatre session. These checks are the responsibility of the anaesthetist and must not be delegated to other personnel. In the event of a change of anaesthetist during and operating session, the checked status of the anaesthetic machine must be agreed.

Before using any anaesthetic apparatus, ventilator, breathing system, or monitor, it is essential to be fully familiar with it. This familiarisation process which may entail study of the instruction manual, is particularly important when faced with new equipment and should be regarded as an essential part of the safety check. Similarly, a thorough understanding must be gained of any equipment assembled in an unfamiliar configuration.

A. Anaesthetic machine
Check that the anaesthetic machine and relevant ancillary equipment are connected to the mains electricity supply (where appropriate) and switched on. Careful note should be taken of any information or labelling on the anaesthetic machine which might refer to its current status.

B. Oxygen analyser
1. *The oxygen analyser should be placed where it can monitor the composition of gases leaving the common gas outlet.*
2. *The analyser should be switched on, checked and calibrated according to the manufacturer's instructions.*

Published in March 1997 by The Association of Anaesthetists of Great Britain and Ireland and reproduced with their permission.

C. Medical gas supplies

1. *Identify and take note of the gases which are being supplied by pipeline, confirming with a 'tug test' that each pipeline is correctly inserted into the appropriate gas supply terminal.*
2. *Check that the anaesthetic apparatus is connected to a supply of oxygen and that an adequate reserve of oxygen is available from a spare cylinder.*
3. *Check that adequate supplies of any other gases intended for use are available and connected as appropriate. All cylinders should be securely seated and turned off after checking their contents.*
   Carbon dioxide cylinders should not normally be present on the anaesthetic machine. A blanking plug should be fitted to any empty cylinder yoke.
4. *All pressure gauges for pipelines connected to the anaesthetic machine should indicate 400 kPa.*
5. *Check the operation of flowmeters, ensuring that each control valve operates smoothly and that the bobbin moves freely throughout its range without sticking. With only the oxygen flow control valve open and a flow of approximately 5 litres per minute, check that the oxygen analyzer display approaches 100%. Turn off all flow control valves.*
6. *Operate the emergency oxygen bypass control and ensure that flow occurs without significant decrease in the pipeline supply pressure. Confirm that the oxygen analyser display approaches 100% during this test. Ensure that the emergency oxygen bypass control ceases to operate when released.*

D. Vaporizers

1. *Check that the vaporizer(s) for the required volatile agent(s) are fitted correctly to the anaesthetic machine, that any back bar locking mechanism is fully engaged and that the control knobs rotate fully through the full range(s). Ensure that the vaporizer is not tilted.* **Turn off the vaporizers**.
2. *Check that the vaporizer(s) are adequately filled and that the filling port is tightly closed.*
3. (i) *Set a flow of oxygen of 5 litres/min and, with the vaporizer turned off, temporarily occlude the common gas outlet. There should be no leak from any of the vaporizer fitments and the flowmeter bobbin should dip.*
   (ii) *Turn each vaporizer on in turn and repeat this test. There should be no leak of liquid from the filling port.* **After this test, ensure that the vaporizers and flowmeters are turned off**.
   (iii) *Should it be necessary to change a vaporizer at any stage, it is essential to repeat the leak test. Failure to do so is one of the commonest causes of critical incidents.*
   (iv) *Removal of a vaporizer from a machine in order to refill it is not considered necessary.*

E. Breathing system

1. *Check all breathing systems which are to be employed. They should be visually inspected for correct configuration and assembly. All connections within the system and to the anaesthetic machine should be secured by 'push and twist'. Ensure that there are no leaks or obstructions in the reservoir bags or breathing system. A pressure leak test should be performed on the breathing system by occluding the patient end and compressing the reservoir bag. Each breathing system poses separate problems. Each should be checked as appropriate and in particular it is necessary to perform an occlusion test on the inner tube of the Bain-type coaxial system, to ensure that it is correctly attached.*

2. Check that the adjustable pressure limiting 'expiratory' valve can be fully opened and closed.
3. The correct operation of the unidirectional valves in a circle system should be carefully checked.
4. If is it intended to use low fresh gas flows in a circle breathing system, there must be a means to analyse the oxygen concentration in the inspiratory limb. End tidal CO_2 and agent concentration must also be monitored in this situation.

F. Ventilator
1. Check that the ventilator is configured correctly for its use. Ensure that the ventilator tubing is securely attached. Set the controls for use and ensure that adequate pressure is generated during the inspiratory phase.
2. Check that a disconnect alarm is present and functions correctly.
3. Check that the pressure relief valve functions correctly at the set pressure.
4. **Ensure that there is an alternative means to ventilate the patient's lungs in the event of ventilator malfunction.**

G. Scavenging
The anaesthetic gas scavenging system should be switched on and functioning. Ensure that the tubing is attached to the appropriate expiratory port of the breathing system or ventilator.

H. Ancillary equipment
1. All ancillary equipment which may be needed should be present, such as laryngoscopes, intubation aids (intubation forceps, bougies), etc. Ensure that all sizes of face masks, airways, tracheal tubes and connectors are available.
2. Check that all laryngoscopes are working.
3. The suction apparatus must be functioning and all connections should be secure; test for the rapid development of an adequate negative pressure.
4. Check that the patient trolley, bed or operating table can be rapidly tilted head-down.

I. Monitoring
1. Ensure that the appropriate monitoring equipment is present, switched on and calibrated.
2. Set all necessary alarm limits, as appropriate.

The Association of Anaesthetists of Great Britain and Ireland cannot be held responsible for failure of an anaesthetic machine as a result of a defect not revealed by these procedures.

Recommendations for Standard of Monitoring during Anaesthesia and Recovery

These guidelines are universally accepted to be the minimum safe practice.

SUMMARY

1. *The Association of Anaesthetists of Great Britain and Ireland strongly recommends that the standard of monitoring used during general anaesthesia should be uniform in all circumstances irrespective of the duration of anaesthesia or the location of administration.*
2. *An anaesthetist must be present throughout the conduct of general anaesthesia.*
3. *Monitoring should be commenced before induction and continued until the patient has recovered from the effects of anaesthesia.*
4. *These recommendations also apply to the administration of local anaesthesia, regional analgesia or sedation where there is a risk of unconsciousness or cardiovascular or respiratory complications.*
5. *A pulse oximeter and capnometer must be available for every patient.*
6. *It is strongly recommended that clinical observation of the patient should be supplemented by continuous monitoring devices displaying heart rate, pulse volume or arterial pressure, oxygen saturation, the electrocardiogram and expired carbon dioxide concentration. Devices for measuring intravascular pressures, body temperature and other parameters should be used when appropriate. It is useful to have both waveform and numerical displays.*
7. *Intermittent non-invasive arterial pressure measurement must be recorded regularly if invasive monitoring is not indicated. If neuromuscular blocking drugs are used a means of assessing neuromuscular function should be available.*
8. *Additional monitoring may be required in certain situations. These recommendations may be extended at any time on the judgement of the anaesthetist.*
9. *A printed record of monitoring measurements provides a contemporaneous record during emergency situations and allows the anaesthetist to concentrate on managing the patient.*
10. *When handing over to recovery staff, anaesthetists should issue clear instructions concerning monitoring during postoperative care. Monitoring of oxygen saturation is strongly recommended for all patients, and temperature monitoring is recommended for patients at risk of hypothermia.*
11. *Standards of monitoring during transfer of sedated, anaesthetised or unconscious patients should be as high as during the administration of anaesthesia. All patients should have oxygen saturation, electrocardiogram and arterial pressure monitored. Other monitors may be appropriate in certain circumstances.*
12. *For interhospital transfers, a specialist retrieval team based at the receiving hospital can have advantages.*

Published in July 1994 by The Association of Anaesthetists of Great Britain and Ireland and reproduced with their permission.

Anaesthetic Record Set

This document outlines recommendations for standard minimum information to be included in an anaesthetic record.

PREOPERATIVE INFORMATION

Patient identity: name, i.d no, date of birth.

Assessment and risk factors: date of assessment, assessor, where assessed, weight (kg), [height(m) optional] basic vital signs (BP HR), medication (incl. contraceptive drugs), allergies, addiction (alcohol, tobacco, drugs), previous GAs, family history, potential airway problems, prostheses, teeth, crowns, investigations, cardiorespiratory fitness, other problems, ASA +/– comment.

Urgency: scheduled (listed on a routine list), urgent (resuscitated, not on a routine list), emergency (not fully resuscitated).

PREOPERATIVE INFORMATION

Checks: nil by mouth, consent, premedication (type and effect).

Place and time: place, date, start and end times.

Personnel: all anaesthetists named, operating surgeon, qualified assistant present, duty consultant informed.

Operation planned/performed.

Apparatus: check performed, anaesthetic room, theatre.

Vital signs recording/charting: monitors used and vital signs (specify).

Drugs and fluids: dose, concentration, volume, cannulation, injection site(s), time and route, warmer used, blood loss, urine output.

Airway and breathing system: route, system used, ventilation: type and mode, airway type, size, cuff, shape, special procedures, humidifier, filter, throat pack, difficulty.

Regional anaesthesia: consent, block performed, entry site, needle used, aid to location, catheter: y/n.

Patient position and attachments: thrombosis prophylaxis, temperature control, limb positions.

Published in April 1996 by The Royal College of Anaesthetists, The Association of Anaesthetists of Great Britain and Ireland, and The Society for Computing and Technology in Anaesthesia and reproduced with their permission.

POSTOPERATIVE INSTRUCTIONS

Drugs, fluids doses, analgesic techniques, special airway instructions, including oxygen, monitoring.

Untoward events: *abnormalities, critical incidents, pre-op, per-op, postoperative, context, cause, effect.*

Hazard flags: *warnings for future care.*

Controlled Drugs

This report gives guidance on the storage, issue and disposal of controlled drugs as relevant to the anaesthetist.

The Medicines Act 1968 controls all aspect of production and distribution of medicinal products. Under the act, medicines may be licensed, special or prepared.

- A **product licence** is granted to a product when the Medicines Control agency is satisfied as to its safety and efficacy for a given indication. It specifies the nature of the drug, pharmaceutical form, strength and packaging.
- The **manufacturer's licence** entitles the holder to manufacture medicinal products.
- **Specials** are medicinal products which have no product licence, but are made by a holder of a manufacturer's licence to order of a clinician. They are supplied on a named patient basis, and the clinician bears responsibility for all aspects of safety.
- **Prepared medicines** have no product licence but are made up in accordance with a prescription under supervision of a pharmacist, who has no manufacturer's licence.
- Many drugs are supplied as licensed products but require dilution or reconstitution, whereupon they become prepared medicines.
- Supply of patient-controlled analgesia syringes should be, in order of preference, licensed where available, failing that a special, failing that a prepared medicine made in a hospital pharmacy.

ISSUE OF CONTROLLED DRUGS IN THE OPERATING DEPARTMENT

- The Misuse of Drugs Regulations (1985) place the responsibility for possession of controlled drugs with the most senior registered nurse on duty, regardless of whether or not he or she has delegated control of access (i.e. key holding) to another nurse or doctor.
- The senior nurse is responsible for ordering, receiving, checking, recording and storing stock; recording the amounts issued to doctors; and returning unused ampoules to stock.
- The doctor is responsible for signing the register, recording the amount administered in the patient notes or anaesthetic record, returning unopened ampoules, and disposing of unused drug in an open ampoule or syringe.
- The pharmacist is responsible for supply to each stock location, regular audit of policies and checking stocks once every 1–3 months.

MULTIPLE DOSING

Except in the case of ampoules designated for multiple use, the association condemns the practice of sharing the contents of an ampoule between patients. This is based on the risks of cross-infection and theft.

Published in October 1995 by The Association of Anaesthetists of Great Britain and Ireland.

PATIENT-CONTROLLED ANALGESIA

- 'Licensed' or 'prepared' solutions are preferred as they are more likely to be sterile and clearly labelled.
- Patient-controlled analgesia and epidural solutions should be supplied in individually sealed bags, and accounted for in the same way as other controlled drugs.

DISPOSAL OF CONTROLLED DRUGS

Controlled drugs cease to be classified as such when rendered unusable or irretrievable. Syringes containing controlled drugs should be emptied before being discarded. Solutions containing controlled drugs should not be disposed of down the sink without the consent of the local water authority. Disposal on to some absorbent material is recommended. There is no legal requirement to record disposal of small quantities of controlled drugs, but local policies may dictate this.

HIV and Other Blood-borne Viruses: Guidance for Anaesthetists

This is the second in the series of association publications on HIV/HBV. It gives information relevant to prevention and management of occupational transmission.

INTRODUCTION

Several factors have made it necessary to review the advice published in 'AIDS and Hepatitis B: guidelines for anaesthetists'. The number of cases of occupational transmission has increased and there is evidence that recommended precautions are not widely observed.

EPIDEMIOLOGY OF HIV AND HBV

HIV

The number of reported cases of acquired immunedeficiency syndrome (AIDS) continues to rise. A total of 5894 cases were reported by April 1992, 3686 of whom have died. The number of individuals who are human immunodeficiency virus (HIV)- positive is not known, but is probably around 50 000.

HBV

Hepatitis B virus (HBV) infection is a major problem throughout the world. In Britain, 2000 cases per year are reported, but many cases are asymptomatic and go unreported.

Following an acute illness, 5–10% of infected adults develop the carrier state, defined as the persistence of hepatitis B surface antigen in the circulation for more than 6 months. One in 500 adults are carriers.

The presence of the 'e' antigen (HBeAg) is associated with the presence of infectious virus, and such patients are a high risk for occupational transmission.

TRANSMISSION AND OCCUPATIONAL EXPOSURE

HIV is transmitted by blood, sexual contact and transplacentally. Other body fluids are designated high risk: amniotic fluid, pericardial fluid, pleural fluid, synovial fluid, cerebrospinal fluid (CSF), peritoneal fluid, semen and vaginal secretions. Faeces, nasal secretions, sputum, saliva, sweat, urine and vomitus are not high risk unless visibly contaminated with blood.

Published in December 1992 by The Association of Anaesthetists of Great Britain and Ireland.

HBV may be present in all body fluid, but transmission has only firmly been attributed to blood, semen and vaginal secretions.

Anaesthetists are at risk of occupational transmission by needle stick injury or contamination of an open wound. The risk of seroconversion for HIV after percutaneous injury was shown to be 0.39%. The risk for hepatitis B transmission is 5–30%.

SCREENING

Screening patients for HIV does not reduce the risk of occupational exposure and cannot be sanctioned without the patient's consent.

PRECAUTIONS

Precautions against occupational transmission must be adopted as a routine part of anaesthetic practice.

- Gloves should be worn during induction, intravenous cannulation and airway manoeuvres. Plastic apron, mask and eye protection should be worn where substantial spillage is likely. Equipment and other articles should not be handled with contaminated gloves.
- Needles should not be resheathed or handed from one person to another. They should be disposed of in a 'sharps' bin.
- Cuts and abrasions on the anaesthetist's skin should be covered with a waterproof dressing.
- Parts of the breathing system outside the patient do not constitute a risk, unless contaminated with blood.
- Non-disposable contaminated equipment should be autoclaved where possible or else thoroughly washed before being left in 2% glutaraldehyde or similar.
- Floors contaminated with blood should be washed in hypochlorite solution.

RESUSCITATION AND INTENSIVE CARE

Although there are no reported cases of transmission during resuscitation, the risk exists. Expired air resuscitation should be performed through a protective device. Gloves and aprons should be available with resuscitation equipment, but resuscitation should not be delayed to meet these requirements.

HIV testing is required to establish the suitability of a patient for organ donation. Although consent cannot be obtained from a ventilated patient, the issue should be discussed with the relatives, and counselling offered where necessary.

The decision to withhold treatment from a patient who is HIV-positive should only be made after full consultation with medical and nursing staff caring for that patient.

PROTECTION AGAINST HBV

All anaesthetists should be immunised against HBV. Those who do not mount adequate antibody responses should receive anti-HBV immunoglobulin in the event of an inoculation injury.

POST-EXPOSURE MANAGEMENT

Following inoculation injury, the puncture should be encouraged to bleed, and the wound washed thoroughly with soap and water. Splashes to the eye or mouth should be irrigated with water.

Any incident must be recorded, and an accident form sent to the unit's manager.

Staff should identify a medical advisor to consult in the event of occupational exposure. Contact should be made within an hour of exposure, if possible. Further action may involve investigation of the HIV/HBV status of the patient involved and, if necessary, adoption of protective measures such as immunoglobulin, AZT, antibiotics, etc.

THE ANAESTHETIST WITH HIV INFECTION

Anaesthetists who suspect they may be infected should seek appropriate testing and advice.

Most opportunistic infections associated with HIV infection are not readily transmitted between individuals. Exceptions are tuberculosis, shingles and salmonellosis. All these produce early symptoms.

HIV encephalopathy is unlikely to present in an anaesthetist still otherwise well enough to work.

The risk of transmission from doctor to patient exists, but it is small. The Health Department has recognised that a risk of transmission exists during 'invasive procedures', defined as surgical entry into tissues, cavities or organs or repair of major traumatic injuries, cardiac catheterisation, obstetric procedures, dental or oral surgery, particularly when injury could occur when the hands are not completely visible. The Health Departments have stated that such procedures should not be performed by infected doctors.

Anaesthetists do not routinely carry out procedures which fall into this category. The HIV-positive anaesthetist may therefore continue to practice provided he/she practices cross-infection precautions routinely, understands the routes of occupational transmission, has sought advice about practice, is familiar with the General Medical Council (GMC) guidance, and is under regular medical supervision.

THE HEPATITIS B-INFECTED ANAESTHETIST

A doctor who is HBeAg- or HBsAg-positive may not perform invasive procedures. Apart from this, an infected anaesthetist may continue in clinical practice.

Blood-borne Viruses and Anaesthesia

Further advice from the Association's blood-borne viruses advisory panel on two specific issues: the new definition of 'exposure-prone procedures' and the transmission of hepatitis C virus via anaesthetic breathing systems.

- The Department of Health (DoH) decided that health care workers infected with HBV or HIV could continue to practice what was defined as 'invasive procedures'. In 1992, the advisory body concluded that anaesthetists did not routinely carry out invasive procedures.
- In 1994, the DoH adopted the term 'exposure-prone procedures' in place of 'invasive procedures', and revised the definition in line with that in North America.
- The full definition of 'exposure-prone procedures' is: 'those procedures where there is a risk that injury to the health worker may result in the exposure of the patient's open tissues to the blood of the worker. These procedures include those where the worker's gloved hand may be in contact with sharp instruments, needle tips or sharp tissues (spicules of bone or teeth) inside a patient's open body cavity, wound or confined anatomical space where the hands or finger tips may not be completely visible at all times'.
- The possibility that an infected anaesthetist could infect a patient by placing fingers in the patient's mouth (for example during insertion of the laryngeal mask airway) was considered. There was no evidence forthcoming to suggest that anaesthetists sustain soft tissue injuries in this way, and it was considered that if such an injury did occur, it would be immediately visible to the anaesthetist. Therefore, the group recommended to council that anaesthesia should **not** be considered an exposure prone specialty. They also recommended that the wearing of gloves be mandatory when placing fingers in a patient's mouth.
- The group also considered a report of a case from Australia in which hepatitis C was transmitted from one patient to four others on the same operating list. It seems likely (though not proven conclusively) that transmission occurred via the anaesthetic breathing system.
- It is known that anaesthetic breathing systems can become contaminated with respiratory tract organisms, and ventilators can cause cross-infection. The incidence of this is unknown, but is liable to increase as a result of increases in multiple resistant tuberculosis, and other factors. Contamination can be reliably prevented only with the use of a pleated hydrophobic membrane filter.
- The group recommended that either an appropriate single-use filter is placed between the patient and the breathing system, or that a new breathing system be used for each patient. Where expired gas sampling is used, the sample should be taken from the breathing system side of the filter.

Update published in January 1996 by The Association of Anaesthetists of Great Britain and Ireland. First edition published in 1988, revised 1992 (see page 52).

Report of the Working Party on Pain After Surgery

A joint Working Party report which comments on the inadequacy of postoperative pain management, and gives recommendations for improvement.

The treatment of pain after surgery in British hospitals has been inadequate and has not advanced significantly for many years. This report describes the background to this persistent failure and makes recommendations to improve the situation.

SUMMARY

The treatment of pain after surgery in the UK is unsatisfactory and evidence in this report points to several ways of improving the situation in all hospitals.

All staff involved in the treatment of postoperative pain should be educated more fully in the areas described in this report and traditional antiquated attitudes should be changed. A patient's pain should not be neglected but assessed and recorded along with other observations such as blood pressure and heart rate. In order to ensure this, it is vital that a named member of staff is responsible for a hospital policy which ensures satisfactory pain relief for all patients after surgery. This activity should be audited and appraised continuously.

The advantages of an acute pain service have been described. This service should be introduced in all major hospitals performing surgery in the UK.

The introduction of new effective and safe methods for providing postoperative pain relief should be encouraged.

The advantages of appropriate facilities in the management of postoperative pain have been described. All major hospitals should have a high dependency unit of sufficient size to support the needs of a modern and effective pain relief policy.

In order to introduce a safe and effective policy, there is a need for properly trained staff and adequate resources.

Research into pain relief after surgery should be encouraged and intensified. There is a need for powerful, safe analgesics and long-acting non-toxic local anaesthetics. If these were available, it is likely that postoperative pain would cease to be a major problem.

There are areas of doubts as to the safety and efficacy of some new methods of analgesia and it is important that research into these techniques should continue. Monitoring of patients to detect undesirable side-effects of analgesic regimens is a major need. The development of inexpensive, easy-to-use monitors to detect the main hazards should be encouraged.

Published in September 1990 by The Royal College of Surgeons of England and The College of Anaesthetists and reproduced with permission from The Royal College of Surgeons of England.

Finally, the use of counselling and psychological methods in the management of postoperative pain is often deficient. These methods may have a useful supportive role and research into this field should be encouraged.

AIMS AND RECOMMENDATIONS

To improve the treatment of postoperative pain in all hospitals by implementation of the following recommendations.

- Improve hospital staff education and challenge traditional attitudes to postoperative pain relief.
- Assess and record pain systematically, involving the patient whenever possible.
- Responsibility for the management of pain relief policy after surgery in each hospital given to a named member of staff.
- Establish acute pain teams in all major hospitals.
- Introduce new methods and utilise existing methods more effectively giving due regard for safety.
- Audit and continuous appraisal of activity.
- Establish appropriate facilities for the provision of adequate postoperative pain relief in all hospitals.
- Provide properly trained staff and resources for these services.

To continue and intensify research into:

- Development of better and safer drugs to relieve pain.
- Monitoring of patients after surgery.
- Safety and efficacy of new methods of pain relief.
- Counselling and psychological methods of pain relief.

Surgical Management of Jehovah's Witnesses

Clinical, legal and ethical issues relating to surgery for Jehovah's Witnesses.

- There are 140 000 Jehovah's Witnesses in the UK and Ireland.
- Jehovah's Witnesses have absolutely refused the transfusion of blood products. They are usually well informed doctrinally, and regarding their right to determine their own treatment.
- It is not the doctor's job to question the beliefs of Jehovah's Witnesses.
- The exact views of each Jehovah's Witness patient should be established, as some forms of transfusion may be acceptable.
- Organ transplantation is acceptable to Jehovah's Witnesses.
- To administer blood against a patient's wishes is unlawful.
- The clinician should decide whether he or she is willing to accept these limitations in management and, if not, refer the patient for further opinion.
- In the management of trauma, the Jehovah's Witness status of a patient may be unknown, although the majority now carry advance directives. In the absence of such a directive, a doctor's clinical judgement should override the opinion of relatives.
- In the case of children of Jehovah's Witnesses, the surgeon should make use of the law to protect the child's interests. In England and Wales, a *Specific Issue Order* may be applied for, to allow transfusion in this situation.
- If a child needs blood in an emergency, it should be given. Failure to do so may leave the surgeon open to criminal prosecution.
- Although children under 16 can give consent to medical treatment if they understand the issues involved, the courts have been willing to overrule refusal of specific procedures by children.
- The High Court is the most appropriate forum for any hearing.

SURGICAL POLICY

- Operations should be carried out by senior members of a team sensitive to the beliefs of Jehovah's Witnesses.
- Any surgery must be preceded by full discussion with the patient, in the presence of a witness, establishing rules of management. A special consent form is available.
- For adult Jehovah's Witnesses, refusal of blood must be honoured.
- For trauma victims identified as Jehovah's Witnesses but lacking documentation, every effort to avoid blood transfusion should be made, but the decision to transfuse should be based on clinical judgement.

Published in 1996 by The Royal College of Surgeons of England.

SPECIAL CONSIDERATIONS IN CHILDREN

Where transfusion is unlikely to be necessary, surgery may proceed in the normal way, and the parents can sign the appropriate forms to show their objection to blood transfusion. The surgeon may choose to say "I will not let your child die for want of a blood transfusion". Every effort should be made to respect the family's wishes, but the well-being of the child is paramount.

SURGICAL TECHNIQUES

Considerations should include:

- minimising blood samples taken for investigation
- the use of iron replacement, erythropoietin, controlled preoperative hypotension and regional anaesthesia
- meticulous attention to haemostasis
- policies on blood substitutes and artificial oxygen transporters
- the acceptability of blood salvage and haemodilution techniques
- cardio-pulmonary bypass without haematogenous priming solutions
- Jehovah's Witnesses maintain a network of hospital liaison committees (Watch Tower: 0181 906 2211).

Report of the Working Party on the Management of Patients with Major Injuries

A report which comments on the inadequacies of trama management, and gives recommendations for improvement.

SUMMARY

1. *The Royal College of Surgeons considers that injury and its consequences rank as the most important health problems of today. The College recommends that the prevention and management of injury should receive greater attention from the government, the Department of Health, the Universities and the research councils.*
2. *The retrospective study undertaken for this report reveals significant deficiencies in the management of seriously injured patients. The prospective studies confirm this finding and, additionally, show positive benefits from consultant involvement at the time of hospital admission.*
3. *The majority of injured patients should be managed, as at present, in large district general hospitals with a wide range of facilities and experienced supporting staff and a Accident and Emergency Department under the supervision of consultants in emergency medicine.*
4. *There should be only one hospital with an A&E department in each NHS district. Other A&E services in the same district should be closed or their freedom to treat the injured restricted.*
5. *Patients with life-threatening injury beyond the facilities or capabilities of a district general hospital should be transferred by high quality transport to a Trauma Centre established at regional or multidistrict level.*
6. *Trauma Centres should provide a 24 hour a day service from consultants in general and orthopaedic surgery, anaesthesia and emergency medicine, and their supporting staff, all of whom should be resident in the hospital during their time on duty. Consultants in other relevant specialties such as cardiothoracic surgery, neurosurgery, and radiology should be immediately available.*
7. *A number of consultant general, orthopaedic and neurosurgeons and anaesthetists should be encouraged to take a major interest in accident surgery but their activities should not be confined to the management of injury. Their training, together with the training of others interested in the management of major injury, should in the future take place in Trauma Centres in this country and overseas.*
8. *Pre-hospital care should be provided by specially trained ambulancemen. In addition to a higher level of therapeutic skills they should be trained in injury severity assessment in order that patients can be conveyed to appropriate hospitals. There should be increased medical involvement in the organisation and training of the ambulance service.*
9. *Radiocommunications between ambulances and the receiving hospitals should be improved.*
10. *Consideration should be given to increasingly sophisticated methods of transport such as helicopters for transfer of patients between hospitals. However, their general introduction*

Published in November 1988 by The Royal College of Surgeons of England and reproduced with their permission.

and use for primary collection of injured patients should only be allowed following an independent assessment of their value.

11. *Standards of Hospital care of the injured should be monitored through a national audit scheme such as the Major Trauma Outcome Study.*

12. *There should be increased emphasis in both undergraduate and postgraduate curricula of the problems and management of the injured.*

13. *Research investment into causes, prevention and management of injury should be dramatically increased.*

14. *The Department of Health and Regional and District Health Authorities should review their policies for the management of the seriously injured patient in the light of the findings and recommendations in this report.*

Recommendations for the Transfer of Patients with Acute Head Injuries to Neurosurgical Units

Clinical, logistic and educational advice on transfer of head-injured patients from district hospitals to neurosurgical centres.

SUMMARY AND RECOMMENDATIONS

1. *There should be a designated consultant in the referring hospital with overall responsibility for the transfer of patients with head injuries to the neurosurgical unit and one at the neurosurgical unit with overall responsibility for receiving the transfers.*
2. *Local guidelines on the transfer of patients with head injuries should be drawn up between the referring hospital trusts and the neurosurgical unit which should be consistent with established national guidelines. Details of the transfer of the responsibility for patient care should also be agreed.*
3. *Thorough resuscitation and stabilisation of the patient must be completed before transfer to avoid complications during the journey. A patient persistently hypotensive, despite resuscitation, must not be transported until all possible causes of the hypotension have been identified and the patient stabilised.*
4. *Only in exceptional circumstances should a patient with a significantly altered conscious level requiring transfer for neurosurgical care not be intubated.*
5. *Patients with head injuries should be accompanied by a doctor with at least 2 years' experience in an appropriate specialty (usually anaesthesia). Ideally, they should be on a specialist register. They should be familiar with the pathophysiology of head injury, the drugs and equipment they will use, working in the confines of an ambulance (or helicopter if appropriate) and have received supervised training in the transfer of patients with head injuries. They must have an adequately trained assistant. They must be provided with appropriate clothing for the transfer, medical indemnity and personal insurance.*
6. *The transfer team must be provided with a means of communication with their base hospital and the neurosurgical unit during the transfer – a portable phone may be suitable.*
7. *Education training and audit are crucial to improving standards of transfer; appropriate time and funding should be provided.*

Published in December 1996 by The Neuroanaesthesia Society of Great Britain and Ireland and The Association of Anaesthetists of Great Britain and Ireland and reproduced with permission from The Association of Anaesthetists of Great Britain and Ireland.

Anaesthesia for ECT

This is based on a section taken from a much larger document entitled 'ECT Handbook' which gives comprehensive guidance on all aspects of electroconvulsive therapy.

Anaesthesia for electroconvulsive therapy (ECT) should be given by someone capable of managing its potential complications in a setting which may be away from the main hospital. The minimum requirement is probably 1 year of anaesthetic experience together with specific instruction by an experienced consultant. Continuity of care is important for patients having a course of treatment. There should be one person to help the anaesthetist and one to recover each patient who has not regained consciousness. The anaesthetist should be aware of the patient's status under the Mental Health Act 1983.

ASSESSMENT OF PATIENTS BEFORE ECT

History and examination should cover:

1. Cardiovascular system: profound haemodynamic changes accompany ECT.
2. Respiratory system: ECT may be hazardous in severe chest disease.
3. Dentition.
4. Obesity or hiatus hernia.
5. Arthritis in jaw or neck.
6. Previous anaesthetic history, medication, drug allergies.

INVESTIGATIONS

1. Full blood count: all patients.
2. Sickle status: Afro-Caribbean, Middle Eastern, Asian and Eastern Mediterranean patients.
3. Urea and electrolytes: in patients on diuretic, or lithium, or with dehydration, renal, cardiac or liver disease.
4. Urinalysis: all patients.
5. Blood sugar: diabetics.
6. Chest X-ray if signs of cardiorespiratory disease.
7. ECG for cardiovascular disease or hypertension.
8. Physical illness should be controlled where possible; in particular dehydration (which decreases the efficacy of ECT) should be corrected.
9. Unfit patients should be refused treatment only after consultation with senior staff. The illness and alternative treatments all carry a mortality. It may be appropriate to treat some high risk patients in the main hospital.

Published in January 1995 by the Special Committee on ECT of The Royal College of Psychiatrists.

CONTRAINDICATIONS.

There are few absolute contraindications:

1. Avoid in phaeochromocytoma; undesirable in severe cardiovascular disease. Treatment should not be carried out within 3 months of a myocardial infarction.
2. Thrombophlebitis, because of the risk of embolisation; treatment may be given once the patient is anticoagulated.
3. Active respiratory tract infection.
4. Upper airway obstruction.
5. Patients with muscle disease should not be treated away from the main hospital.
6. Undesirable in patients with untreated intracranial aneurysm, or within 3 months of a stroke.
7. Raised intracranial pressure.
8. Acute closed angle glaucoma.

However:

- Old age alone is not a contraindication.
- ECT is safe with pacemakers. The patient should be isolated from the ground and ECG monitored.
- Patients with COAD can be treated if their respiratory function is optimised.
- Patients with cerebral tumours can be treated provided intracranial pressure is not raised.

INDUCTION AGENTS

Intravenous induction is the norm. All agents reduce seizure duration to some extent.

Methohexitone is the drug of choice in a dose of 0.75–0.9 mg/kg. Higher doses reduce seizure duration and increase postictal amnesia. Lignocaine can reduce pain on injection without affecting seizure duration.

Thiopentone produces similar seizure duration. It increases cardiac dysrhythmias two- to fourfold, compared with methohexitone.

Diazepam has been recommended (in 1975), but has many disadvantages.

Etomidate produces similar seizure characteristics to methohexitone. The adrenal effects might preclude use for repeated anaesthesia.

Despite its advantages, propofol reduces seizure duration by 40%, and is probably contraindicated.

MUSCLE RELAXANTS

Relaxants are used to prevent injury, without ablating signs of muscle activity. Suxamethonium is first choice in a dose of 0.5 mg/kg. Seizure duration is inversely proportional to suxamethonium dose. The duration of action of suxamethonium is reduced by ECT, and slightly prolonged by lithium therapy. Suxamethonium myalgia occurs in only 2% of cases. Mivacurium is probably the best alternative where suxamethonium is contraindicated.

VENTILATION

All patients should receive oxygen before the ECT stimulus. Hypoxia does not augment treatment. Seizure duration can be increased by hyperventilation (for example a 68% increase when the alveolar CO_2 was reduced from 5 to 2 kPa).

ANAESTHETIC AND MONITORING EQUIPMENT

The anaesthetist must have adequately trained assistance during ECT treatment. All staff should have training and regular updating in basic and advanced life support. The responsibility for keeping equipment in working order should be clearly defined.

All patients should be anaesthetised on a tipping trolley. A complex anaesthetic machine is probably not necessary; oxygen and suction are essential. Nitrous oxide and volatile agents are not necessary. A ventilator is not required.

The best monitor is a pulse oximeter. Capnography must be available. ECG is less practical for routine use but should be available.

An emergency drug box should be available, containing diazemuls, aminophylline, salbutamol, hydrocortisone, adrenaline, atropine, lignocaine, isoprenaline, verapamil, esmolol, nitrates, naloxone, dantrolene and 50% dextrose. A means of measuring blood glucose, a chest drain set and central venous pressure lines should be available.

RECOVERY

The recovery area must be of an appropriate size, with appropriate monitoring and resuscitation equipment. There should be one staff member for each patient not in control of protective reflexes. The anaesthetist and psychiatrists must remain within easy reach of the recovery area.

Assistance for the Anaesthetist

Standards for provision and training of operating department assistants and anaesthetic nurses.

SUMMARY

1. *The safe administration of anaesthesia necessitates skilled and exclusive assistance. Anaesthetists must not tolerate the continuation of unsafe working practices, particularly if they involve trainees.*
2. *The current means by which help is provided for anaesthetists are failing nationally to achieve consistently acceptable numbers or quality of staff. This has already led to curtailment of elective surgery. Therefore, the problem must be solved if anaesthetic services are to be maintained.*
3. *Assistance must be provided by staff who have been specially trained, and who have acquired relevant skills, working within a structure that promotes proper management, pay and working conditions.*
4. *Nurse and ODA training are both adequate foundations on which such further training can be based.*
5. *Proposals are described which would replace, and significantly improve, current assistance arrangements.*
6. *Suitably qualified staff will be either Anaesthetic Department Nurses (ADNs) or Anaesthetic Department Assistants (ADAs)*
7. *The ENB course no. 182 provides appropriate training for nurses. ADA status will be achieved by ODAs who satisfy competence-based assessment linked to the National Council for Vocational Qualifications (NCVQ).*

Published in November 1988 by the Association of Anaesthetists of Great Britain and Ireland and reproduced with their permission.

Anaesthesia in Great Britain and Ireland: A Physician-only Service

Outlines the Association's views on some aspects of the manpower shortage in anaesthesia, with particular reference to the issue of non-physician anaesthetists.

- Hospital-based anaesthesia in Great Britain and Ireland is exclusively a medical specialty. A number of factors have led to a serious consultant manpower shortage within the specialty. This situation poses a threat to the provision of safe anaesthetic practice in the UK.
- Although it is not legally necessary to be medically qualified to dispense medical treatment, it is essential that the patient is aware of the status of the person providing that treatment. Doctors have a continuing duty of care, and a responsibility to ensure the competence of any individual to which they delegate care. The GMC has stated that a doctor is forbidden to enable anyone not registered with the GMC to carry out tasks that require the knowledge and skills of a doctor.
- If a known incompetent person causes harm while caring for a patient, the delegating anaesthetist is liable to be charged with gross professional misconduct.
- The cost of employing nurse anaesthetists has been simplistically assumed to be low, on the basis that in other countries they earn on average half that of a physician. This ignores many important factors, such as the restrictions on nurses' hours of work, the cost of implementing a training course, the added cost of physician supervision and the negative effect that nurse anaesthesia has on theatre efficiency and turnover. Indemnity cover may also be expensive, and if physician anaesthetists are to be used to train nurse anaesthetists, then this will reduce their availability for service provision.
- Studies of mortality from anaesthesia in countries with non-physician anaesthesia show interesting differences from our own national reports.
- The Association believes that the role of the anaesthetic assistant needs to be reassessed. There are many routine tasks performed by anaesthetists which could equally well be done by other suitably trained staff, allowing anaesthetists to use their skills more effectively.
- Much can be done to improve the efficiency of operating lists.
- There is a lack of recognition for the activities of anaesthetists outside the operating theatre, and many workload plans ignore legitimate consultant absences.

CONCLUSIONS

The Association believes that the introduction of non-physician anaesthetists, would not solve any of the current problems, and would create new ones, such as potential

Published in March 1996 by The Association of Anaesthetists of Great Britain and Ireland.

changes in patient safety levels, postoperative morbidity, training considerations, increased costs and potential medico-legal problems.

RECOMMENDATIONS

- Optimum patient care of patients is a fundamental tenet of NHS practice. It can often best be achieved by adopting a 'team approach' which efficiently utilises a blend of the skills of doctors, nurses and other professionals. This needs to be further explored.
- Anaesthesia in Great Britain and Ireland should continue as a physician-administered specialty.
- The provision of skilled assistance for the anaesthetists should be reassessed. This assistance must be of high standard and dedicated to anaesthesia.
- The efficiency of operating theatre scheduling must be improved. The Anaesthetic Directorate is fundamental in the efficient running of the operating theatre.
- Consultant staffing levels need to take account of 'achieving a balance' (see page 141), junior doctors' hours legislation and the structured training programmes need to be attained.
- Regular revision of manpower requirements is necessary to avoid future crises in manpower provision in anaesthesia.

Consultant–Trainee Relationships: A Guide for Consultants

Good practice guide for consultants with respect to their relationship with trainees in their department.

SUMMARY OF RECOMMENDATIONS

1. *Consultants must accept responsibility for the welfare of their trainees.*
2. *Departments of anaesthesia should have a common room.*
3. *Departments of anaesthesia should appoint personal mentors.*
4. *Trainees should not undertake clinical duties without adequate rest.*
5. *The recommendations of CEPOD should be studied by all consultants with trainee responsibility.*
6. *The needs of overseas doctors should be recognised and met.*
7. *The trainee should register with a general practitioner on taking up a post.*
8. *The departmental secretary should be acknowledged to have an important role.*
9. *Every department should have a handbook of information.*
10. *Counselling must be available to trainees.*

Published in May 1989 by The Association of Anaesthetists of Great Britain and Ireland and reproduced with their permission.

NHS (Appointment of Consultants) Regulations 1996 Good Practice Guide

Regulations governing the consultant appointment process.

VACANCY/ESTABLISHMENT OF THE POST

Planning the post
Employing bodies should plan consultant appointments well in advance. All posts should be available to job sharers. A job description should be prepared.

Preparation of a job description
- Initially, the job description is prepared locally, with information on the employing body, commitments and the range of services offered.
- The Regional Adviser of the Royal College or Faculty should have the opportunity to comment on the draft job description.
- When in doubt, the Regional Adviser should discuss his concerns with the medical director of the trust.
- If there is disagreement, The Royal College should be involved as mediator. Where agreement cannot be reached, the College should explain the implications of this in terms of training recognition, and this information should be available to all applicants.
- Where the post will involve significant undergraduate teaching, it is good practice to forward the job description to the Dean of the relevant medical school.

Selection criteria
- Employers should prepare selection criteria, and outline the minimum requirements in a manner that avoids discrimination. Applicants should have access to copies of these criteria.
- Specialist registrars will be able to apply for consultant jobs within 3 months of being admitted to the GMC's specialist register.

Advertising the post
- All posts must be advertised, unless permission not to has been obtained from the Secretary of State.
- Advertisements should appear in at least two nationally distributed journals.
- Advertisements should encourage applications from both sexes and all sections of the community.

Published in March 1996 by the NHS Executive.

THE ADVISORY APPOINTMENTS COMMITTEE (AAC)

Selecting the AAC
The date for the AAC should be arranged before advertising, and should be about 6 weeks after the closing date.

Membership
- Core membership consists of:
    - a lay member (normally the chair of the employing authority or another non-executive director)
    - an external assessor from the college
    - the chief executive (or senior manager)
    - the Medical director (or medically qualified nominee)
    - a consultant, usually from the relevant specialty
    - A university representative, for posts with teaching or research commitments.
- Other members may be added, for example when the post covers more than one body.
- The AAC should not contain a close relative of a candidate, nor consist entirely of men nor entirely of women. The retiring consultant should not be a member.

The function of the AAC
The AAC decides which, if any, candidate is suitable and recommends him/her for appointment. The AAC may not recommend a candidate it has not interviewed. Candidates may be considered *in absentia,* and if they are deemed most suitable, the AAC must be reconvened to interview that candidate.

The Chair's role
- The Chair should ensure that members consider candidates on professional merit, and act in accordance with anti-discrimination legislation.
- The Chair should ensure that members declare any interest they have in a candidate, for example if they have given a reference.

The role of other members
- All members should have received training in shortlisting and interviewing, especially with respect to equal opportunities and personal matters which must not be discussed at interview.
- Selection is based purely on qualifications, experience and other qualities necessary for the post. Members should keep contemporaneous records of proceedings, including their reasons for accepting or rejecting candidates. Courts or Industrial Tribunals may question the Committee, and may wish to see such notes.
- In any other context, the proceedings are confidential.

THE PRE-INTERVIEW PROCESS

- Applicants will be supplied with an information package. They will be asked to complete an application form, and a CV. The applicant should not be asked to provide multiple copies of applications.

- Employing bodies should ensure ethnic and gender monitoring. A nominated manager shall make an initial check on the basic information given by candidates.
- Copies of all applications are sent to the AAC for consideration.
- Each member of the committee must have the opportunity to contribute to selection of candidates. Short-listing must be carried out against selection criteria.
- The college assessor can advise on whether those in specialist registrar posts are likely to complete a training programme successfully.
- Before interviews, the Committee should draw up objective criteria against which to consider the candidates.
- The health questionnaire is confidential and only opened after a candidate is recommended for appointment.
- References should be taken up when the candidates are invited for interview.

The interviews
- The Chair should ensure that candidates are questioned according to the principles of equal opportunities, and that candidates are not questioned on:
    - the type of contract the applicant would opt for
    - matters relating to terms and conditions or salary
    - whether or not the applicant would undertake private practice.
- Consideration of individual candidates should be made after all the interviews. References are available for consideration, but members should only take account of actual written remarks, not hearsay or third party comment.
- The Chair should work for a unanimous decision, using a vote where this is not possible.
- It is desirable for an officer of the employing body to give advice on terms and conditions, but he/she would not participate in any other way.

THE POST-INTERVIEW PROCESS
- A brief report of the AAC should be prepared and signed by the Chair of the AAC.
- All records should be kept for 6 months.
- The successful candidate should be formally offered the post in writing within 2 working days of the appointment.

GENERAL
- A consultant will usually have independent clinical responsibility for any patient entrusted to his/her care by the employing authority.
- Canvassing for support in applications is prohibited, though preliminary visits are encouraged.
- Applications should be handled so as to safeguard confidentiality.
- In respect of duties involving termination of pregnancy, the employing bodies must conform to guidance in HSG (94)39.

Workload for Consultant Anaesthetists

Workload, duties, contracts, job plans and other issues of relevance to anaesthetists and their employers.

INTRODUCTION

This report updates recommendations in the light of the DoH circular HC(90)16.

WORK PATTERNS

To clarify work patterns the employing authority shall make a general assessment, in terms of notional half days (NHDs) and fractions thereof, in the average time per week required by an average practitioner in the grade and specialty to perform the duties of the posts, **A notional half day is regarded as the equivalent of a period of 3.5 hours flexibly worked**, *and further the duties of the post will be customarily assessed in the flexible way provided for in the terms of service.*

The contract which describes the consultant workload is therefore uniquely defined in NHDs. Thus both job descriptions and job plans must recognise and use these terms.

OPERATING LISTS

An operating list is not the same as an NHD.

DUTIES OF CONSULTANT ANAESTHETISTS

Work is classified as involving fixed or flexible commitments.

Fixed commitments are those which substantially affect the use of other NHS resources. These should number no more than seven NHDs per week.

Flexible commitments include all other activities undertaken on behalf of the NHS. These include:

- associated clinical anaesthetic services, i.e. preoperative and postoperative care. Time allocated for this should be at least one third of the theatre commitment.
- Emergency anaesthetic services. A heavy emergency workload should be reflected in a reduced fixed commitment.
- Resuscitation services.
- Teaching/training/examining/accreditation.
- Research, audit and professional advice.

Published in July 1990 by The Association of Anaesthetists of Great Britain and Ireland and The College of Anaesthetists. The work patterns are reproduced with permission from The Association of Anaesthetists of Great Britain and Ireland.

HONORARY CONTRACT HOLDERS

Flexibility should be allowed in the way in which NHS commitments are fulfilled by academic staff.

CONSULTANTS' MANAGEMENT RESPONSIBILITIES

Authorities may enter into a separate contract for up to two temporary additional NHDs with a consultant who has taken on significant management responsibilities (such as clinical audit, clinical director, or in leadership of the resource management initiative) or with any of his/her colleagues who takes up clinical commitments relinquished by the former.

JOB PLANS

A job plan is a detailed description of the duties and responsibilities of a consultant and of the facilities available to carry them out. They are subject to annual review.

The health authority and the consultant are responsible for agreeing the consultant's duties. The job plan will identify the nature and timing of the consultant's fixed commitments. Except in an emergency, the consultant shall fulfil fixed commitments unless agreed otherwise with the local general manager. Where agreement cannot be reached on proposed amendments to the job plan, the consultant may appeal.

The general manager will initiate discussions on an individual job plan. It is advised that a corporate response should be agreed within the division/directorate, so that the anaesthetic service to the hospital is covered, although each consultant will be individually responsible for agreement of their own job plan.

The general manager may seek advice from the Director of Public Health.

Consultants will not be subject to this arrangement until they have been in the post for 3 years.

CONTRACTS

There are a number of types of contract.

- **Whole-time**: contracted to work for the NHS for substantially the whole of their professional time.
- **Maximum part-time**: also contracted for substantially the whole of their professional time in the NHS, paid 10/11ths of the whole-time salary.
- **Part-time**: contracted with the NHS for up to nine NHDs and paid 1/11th of the whole-time scale per NHD worked.
- **Honorary**: have a remunerative contract with another body, for example a university.

OPTION AGREEMENT

Maximum part-time and whole-time contract holders have the same NHS workload. The option agreement allows the consultant to move between the two contracts without any clinical change in workload, provided they work at least 10 NHDs.

NHDs worked = total number of hours spent at various duties ÷ 3.5.

PRIVATE PRACTICE

Permitted earnings from private practice (i.e. earnings outside category 2) depend on type of contract.

Whole-time consultants can earn up to 10% of gross whole-time salary including distinction awards. At the end of each financial year they must submit a return indicating that their private practice income has not exceeded this level for the year. Fully audited accounts are not normally necessary but may be requested.

Whole-time consultants who exceed this limit 2 years running will automatically be regraded as maximum part-time at the end of the third year, unless by that time they have reduced their private commitments. Once regraded, the consultant may not return to whole-time status until after two consecutive years of earnings below the 10% limit.

There is no limit on the earnings of maximum part-time, or part-time, contract holders. The options for honorary consultants will depend on the agreement with their employing authorities.

DISTINCTION AWARDS

Distinction awards are made by the Secretary of State on advice from a Central Advisory Committee. The criteria for any award must show full commitment to clinical work together with additional items such as development of new techniques, research, teaching, etc.

Awards are made for 5-year periods and are then renewable. They are paid *pro rata* for the number of contracted NHDs.

The criteria for 'C' awards have altered.

NHS TRUSTS

Subject to the passage of necessary legislation, NHS trusts will be responsible for arranging the duties of the consultants they employ, whether under existing contractual provisions or under such arrangements as the parties may agree. It is essential that superannuation arrangements are verified in the event of a change in remuneration.

TRAVELLING TIME

All consultants should include travelling time between hospitals and on emergency call out, and those on part-time and maximum part-time contracts should include travelling between home and hospital up to half an hour each way per day.

Heads of Agreement:
Ministerial Group on Junior Doctors' Hours

The agreed suggestions and recommendations on reducing junior doctors' hours.

GENERAL STATEMENT OF INTENT

All junior doctors must work reasonable hours consistent with the requirements of training. Educational objectives can be met within an maximum average 72-hour week, and the aim is to reduce average contracted hours to this level. In the short term, no junior doctor in a hard-pressed post should be contracted for more than an average of 83 hours per week. Maximum periods of duty should be stated in respect of training posts.

Where application of restrictions causes a gap in service, this must be filled in a manner consistent with 'achieving a balance'. Increases in the number of career grade doctors will be required.

Funding will be required for these changes.

MECHANISMS FOR CHANGE

Working patterns

Where appropriate, shift systems should replace traditional rota arrangements. Where shift systems are not appropriate, working patterns should be altered in other ways, for example time off after a night on duty, reducing the number of tiers of junior cover and/or increasing the use of cross-cover, or employing more part-time staff to improve flexibility.

Consultants' role in providing cover

Expansion of the consultant grade, over and above that required by 'achieving a balance', targeted to areas with particular problems regarding hours is needed.

The Confidential Enquiry into Perioperative Deaths (CEPOD) and other national audits have called for increased supervision by consultants. Any increase in consultant emergency work must be met with an equivalent increase in consultant numbers.

There are three provisos:

1. Performing tasks that are within the competence of other doctors is a waste of consultants' skills.
2. Consultants should not be required to be resident on call.

Published by the Department of Health.

3. The problem of excessive hours should not be transferred from consultants to juniors.

CONFIGURATION OF ON CALL TEAMS

The above measures will result in a range of configurations in the acute specialties, for example:

- consultant, middle grade (on conventional rota), SHO or house officer, probably working a partial shift system
- consultant, SHO (working on a partial shift).

These changes will be facilitated if consultants move towards team-based working, as opposed to the 'firm' system.

CONTRACTUAL ARRANGEMENTS

Current arrangements are not sufficiently flexible to meet the variety of circumstances in which juniors work. This must be changed.

Appropriate duties
Many duties carried out by junior doctors could be performed by non-medical staff.

Educational approval
Educational approval should be withdrawn from training posts in which hours of work and duty are excessive.

Numbers of staff doctors
Staff grade doctors should be deployed flexibly to reduce junior doctors' hours, but inappropriate use of the grade should be prevented.

Distribution of training grade staff
Improved distribution can be used as a means of facilitating reductions in hours.

Allocations of new SHO posts
Posts released following 'achieving a balance' should be targeted in order to facilitate reductions in hours.

Contribution by hospital practitioners and clinical assistants
This possible contribution to reductions in hours should be explored.

Work environment and job descriptions
Recruitment packages for training posts should stress features such as accommodation and support, as well as quality and quantity of experience, training and supervision.

Capital planning and rationalisation of acute services/sites
This would result in reduction of junior doctors' hours.

Task forces
Regional task forces should be established with a remit to examine local areas of difficulty with hours.

Monitoring progress
The ministerial group and its technical group will each meet regularly to ensure progress.

Recommendations for action
The agreement will be implemented in three ways:

1. Health authorities should take immediate action to reduce hours, as suggested in this document.
2. The various parties to the agreement will issue further guidance on a range of issues (see below).
3. Regional task forces should be set up.

The various parties should take the following action:

UK Health Departments should issue the following guidelines:

- on maximum periods of duty, covering the three types of working arrangement (full shift, partial shift, rota)
- on the role of the regional task forces
- on the adoption by nursing, administrative and technical staff of some duties currently carried out by junior doctors
- on good practice regarding job descriptions
- on the implications for capital planning.

They should also:

- consider what extra funding is required
- explore with the profession any scope for increasing the use of clinical assistants.

The Medical Royal Colleges should:

- issue guidance on the particular arrangements for reducing junior doctors' hours in their own specialties.

The Central Consultants and Specialists Committee should:

- issue guidance on the changing role of consultants
- issue guidance on moving to a team-based method of working
- undertake a joint review of the terms and conditions of staff grade appointments, with a view to deploying such doctors more flexibly.

The Hospital Junior Staff Committee should:

- negotiate to secure necessary changes in juniors' contracts to encourage flexible working patterns.

NHS Management should:

- implement further reductions in hours
- redirect resources to enable implementation of this agreement
- locally review the environment of doctors in training.

The 'achieving a balance' technical subgroup should:

• consider the manpower consequences of shift systems
• examine the potential for redistribution of available trainees.

Ministerial Group on Junior Doctors' Hours – Heads of Agreement: Responsibilities of Medical Royal Colleges

> The College's interpretation of agreements on junior doctors' hours and how they apply to the profession of anaesthesia.

GENERAL PRINCIPLES

Anaesthesia is different from other specialties in that:

1. Anaesthetic services are provided by teams of anaesthetists who are required to supply instant response;
2. Where there is no registrar establishment, the consultant is likely to be second on call;
3. Shift systems have existed for years, as anaesthetists have never worked in 'firm' systems.

The College agrees that work should not be simply transferred from juniors to consultants.

GENERAL SOLUTIONS

1. Acute services in each district should be concentrated on one site.
2. The creation of extra consultant posts could allow more surgical work to be carried out during the day.
3. Staff grade anaesthetists can make a useful contribution to the provision of services.
4. Doctors with domestic commitments should be used fully.

COLLEGE GUIDELINES

- The term 'experienced SHO' should be defined. A minimum requirement should be possession of part I F.C.Anaes.
- Cross-cover is not appropriate in anaesthesia, except in intensive care.
- Qualified locums should be available.
- Shifts of work greater than 24 hours are undesirable, but there are advantages to permitting 48-hour weekend shifts. Partial shifts are impractical, and would reduce elective work and affect training.
- No consultant should be first on call or required to sleep in hospital, nor be on call with only an inexperienced SHO.
- A staffed emergency theatre should be available during the day and early evening.
- Higher specialist training (HST) should not be included in intermediate cover. Training may best be managed with a 1 in 3 rota.

Published in April 1991 by The Royal College of Anaesthetists.

Department of Anaesthesia: Secretariat and Accommodation

Standards for the provision of secretarial assistance and office accommodation for departments of anaesthesia.

SECRETARIAL ASSISTANCE

- The departmental secretary is the 'lynch pin' of the system.
- Levels of support staffing depend on the number of consultants in the department, but non-consultant career grades and training staff need access to secretarial assistance, as may other non-medical staff members.
- Other factors to take into account are the clinical services provided, teaching commitments, audit, extra-departmental activities and managerial activities of the clinical directorate.

Requirements

- Core requirements are an office manager and departmental secretary. In small departments, this may be met by an office manager with secretarial skills.
- Extended requirements depend on other services offered:
  - Intensive Therapy Unit (ITU): a four-bed unit with at least 200 admissions per year requires one whole-time equivalent (WTE) medical secretary, responsible to the ITU director.
  - Non-acute pain management: a service running clinics for 3–4 NHDs per week with associated in-patient work, requires one WTE medical secretary.
  - The fully developed clinical directorate may require a business manager, office manager, anaesthetic department secretary, ITU secretary, pain management secretary, operating department support including secretary, information input officer, stores procurement officer, and DSU staff including admissions officer and clerical officer.

DEPARTMENTAL ACCOMMODATION

- The Association strongly commends the guidelines produced by the West Midlands Regional Health Authority entitled 'Planning Guide no. 104: Department of Anaesthesia'.
- For maximum efficiency the department should be a suite of rooms close to operating theatres, ITU, HDU, recovery and A&E.
- Academic departments should be contiguous to the NHS department.
- Planning should take account of the provision of natural light, security and extra floor space of at least 33% for 'circulation space'.
- Communications by a high quality phone system, with or without an intercom to clinical areas, should be provided.

Published in December 1992 by The Association of Anaesthetists of Great Britain and Ireland.

- Space and power supplies should be provided for computer facilities.
- Recommended accommodation, based on a department with 10 WTE consultants, is:
    - general office: for office manager and departmental secretary
    - office: director/chairman
    - office: business manager
    - consultant offices: one for every two WTE consultant anaesthetists
    - senior registrar(s) office: one for every two senior registrars
    - staff lounge: of a size of 3.5 m^2 per consultant, preferably with kitchen area
    - library/quiet room
    - workshop/store/laboratory
    - seminar room
    - computer room/audit office
    - office for pain management secretary
    - locker bay
    - WCs.
- Supplementary accommodation:
    - anaesthetic sister/senior ODA office
    - on call accommodation (if not provided elsewhere)
    - office for ITU secretary
    - cleaner's room.

Efficiency of Theatre Services

Suggestions from a joint Working Group on improving the efficient use of operating theatres.

SUMMARY OF MAIN RECOMMENDATIONS

1. *Theatre services management structure* – a Theatre Director (or equivalent) should be appointed to establish and implement guidelines for theatre utilisation.
2. *Matching beds*, patients and theatre time – close collaboration between the surgical teams and the admitting officer is essential. There should be regular revision of waiting lists.
3. *Urgent and emergency surgery* – the provision of a dedicated theatre is recommended strongly.
4. *Special theatres* – single specialty theatres should be kept to a minimum.
5. *Training and supervision of medical staff* – adequate time for training must be allowed.
6. *List management and anaesthetic assessment* – operating lists should be prepared on the day before surgery to enable proper assessment and optimum list arrangement. Pre-admission clinics are recommended.
7. *Cancellation and under-utilisation of lists* – there must be adequate notice of list cancellation to allow re-allocation of resources. Departures from normal practice should be routinely investigated.
8. *Infected cases* – efficient theatre cleaning procedures should be adopted.
9. *Initial and continuing education of theatre staff* – recruitment and retention of trained nursing staff must be enhanced. Additional training should be encouraged and training budgets protected.
10. *Theatre support staff* – sufficient supporting staff are essential.
11. *Recovery facilities* – a wider role for anaesthetic assistants would offer more flexibility for recovery area staffing.
12. *Data collection systems* – efficient management depends upon the availability of relevant data. Data collection systems may be of value.

Published in September 1989 by The Association of Anaesthetists of Great Britain and Ireland, The Association of Surgeons of Great Britain and Ireland, and The British Orthopaedic Association. Reproduced with permission from The Association of Anaesthetists of Great Britain and Ireland.

Immediate Post-anaesthetic Recovery

Standards for the provision of, and care of patients within, postoperative recovery rooms.

BASIC RECOVERY FACILITIES

Where the anaesthetist is unable to remain with the patient during the immediate post-operative period, accountability for the patient's care must be transferred to trained recovery staff.

Transfer of patients

Patients should normally be transferred to recovery on a tipping trolley in the lateral position. Anaesthetic record, fluid and drug charts should be available. Handover information should include:

- patients name, type of anaesthetic, operation, names of surgeon and anaesthetist
- summary of patient's condition; significant preoperative factors (e.g. deaf mute)
- postoperative orders including oxygen, monitoring, fluid, medications and analgesia.

The anaesthetist should ensure that recovery staff are happy to take responsibility.

If patients remain in recovery after the end of the list, an anaesthetist should be immediately available.

Immediate recovery period

One-to-one nursing is required until the patient is able to maintain his/her own airway. In hospitals with an emergency surgical service, fully staffed recovery facilities must be available at all times.

Patients should remain in recovery with a continuous nursing presence until discharge criteria are met. Discharge is sanctioned by the anaesthetist or a nominated deputy.

Observation and records

The patient should receive continuous clinical observation. The following information should be recorded: time, oxygen administration, oxygen saturation, respiratory rate, heart rate, rhythm, arterial blood pressure, level of consciousness, adequacy of pain relief, sensory level (for regional anaesthesia), intravenous infusions, drugs administered, operation site review, any other monitoring.

In addition, a daily record should be made including patient names, times admitted/discharged and destination.

Published in February 1991 by The Association of Anaesthetists of Great Britain and Ireland.

Administration of drugs

Drugs to be administered should be clearly prescribed. Drugs delivered by infusion should be clearly labelled.

Discharge criteria

- The patient is conscious, can maintain a clear airway, and protective reflexes are present.
- Breathing and oxygenation are satisfactory.
- Cardiovascular system is stable.
- Adequate analgesic and antiemetic provisions are made.
- Temperature is within normal limits.

If respiratory stimulants or vasopressors are used, the patient should not be discharged until the anaesthetist is satisfied that repeat administration will not be required.

Discharge home from recovery

This requires additional criteria.

The patient should be accompanied by an 'adult of suitably robust dimensions', who will remain with the patient for 24 hours.

Advice on analgesia, postoperative information and contact arrangements should be given.

The patient should receive written and verbal warnings against driving, cooking, etc.

THE PURPOSE-BUILT RECOVERY ROOM

The recovery area should be as close to theatres as possible. An area of 1.5 bays per theatre is usually adequate.

Recommended floor space per bay is 9.3 m². Room temperature should be 21–22°C, with a relative humidity of 38–45%. The room's ventilation system should provide 15 air changes per hour. At least one scavenging point should be provided.

Plans for new recovery units should include piped oxygen, nitrous oxide and suction. Each bay should have six 13 A sockets. There should be adequate telephone sockets, sinks and waste bins.

Consideration should be given to the provision of infra-red overhead heaters.

Trolleys

All trolleys should have oxygen cylinders with key, mask and tubing, and a t-piece for a laryngeal mask airway. They should also have suction equipment, padded cot sides, an adjustable back rest, a tilting mechanism operable from the head end, locking steerable wheels, infusion poles, and a tray for notes and equipment.

Bays

Each bay should have oxygen, facemasks (fixed and variable performance), Mapleson 'C' or self-inflating bag, pulse oximeter, ECG monitor, suction, sphygmomanometer, sharps box, airways, bin, vomit bowl and tissues.

Additional equipment

Additional equipment for the unit should include items for paediatric use, an anaesthetic machine with intubation equipment, and miscellaneous items such as thermometers, heating devices and X-ray screen.

Appropriate drugs for routine use and management of emergencies such as cardiac arrest and malignant hyperthermia should be kept in recovery. Access to intravenous fluids and blood products should be readily available.

TRAINING OF RECOVERY STAFF

Training for recovery staff should encompass:

- understanding of anatomy, physiology and pharmacology. Training in airway management and resuscitation. Monitoring requirements and equipment, plus nursing needs of patients in a wide range of specialties. Extra training in specialist units will be required
- a full range of patient groups
- formal assessment on completion of training.

Training in basic operating theatre nursing may improve flexibility.

Regular in-service training should be available. Where appropriate, training in defibrillation, intravenous drug administration, topping up epidurals, assessing level of regional block and preparation and use of patient-controlled analgesia devices should be made available to staff.

Post-basic courses for anaesthetic (ENB 182) and theatre (ENB 183) nursing are satisfactory. Other non-nationally approved courses require careful assessment of content.

The National Vocational Qualification (NVQ) in Operating Theatre Practice at level 3 ensures competence in recovery care, except for the administration of drugs.

Hospitals should develop written guidelines and standards which should be audited regularly.

The High Dependency Unit: Acute Care in the Future

Aspects of the development and management of high dependency units.

SUMMARY

Successful introduction of progressive patient care, whereby a patient moves from one site to another as their clinical condition changes, necessitates wider provision of high dependency care.

INTRODUCTION

In 1988, The Association of Anaesthetists of Great Britain and Ireland commissioned a survey of current practice in general ICUs. The survey revealed that there are few formal high dependency units in the UK, many ICU patients could be nursed more appropriately on an HDU, and that the majority of clinicians recognised that a proportion of general ward patients would benefit from HDU.

A further report has thus been commissioned to indicate why and how high dependency care should be provided.

PROGRESSIVE PATIENT CARE

...may be defined as *'a system of organising patient care in which patients are grouped together in units depending on their need for care as determined by their degree of illness rather than by traditional factors such as medical or surgical specialty. The three usual levels of care are intensive, intermediate, and minimal or self care.'*

DEFINITIONS

- ICU: patients are admitted for treatment of actual or impending organ failure.
- HDU: patients require more intensive observation, treatment and nursing care than can normally be provided on a general ward. It could manage invasive monitoring but not mechanical ventilation.
- Coronary care unit: a place for intensive observation of coronary patients.
- Recovery room: patients are admitted from theatre and discharged when conscious and stable.

There is some overlap in these definitions.

Published in February 1991 by The Association of Anaesthetists of Great Britain and Ireland. The definition of progressive patient care is reproduced with permission from The Association of Anaesthetists of Great Britain and Ireland.

RATIONALE FOR DEVELOPING HIGH DEPENDENCY UNITS

An HDU should make best use of available resources. It should provide an intermediate level of care, maintenance of quality, efficiency and economy.

METHODS OF DELIVERY

High dependency care can be provided with a purpose-built area, or by designating a portion of each general ward and placing the appropriate staff and equipment in that area.

A central location might provide better economy and concentration of expertise. Multiple sites would cause fewer problems of continuity of care, and allow greater flexibility.

The number of beds required could be ascertained with a 6-month audit, considering nursing dependency scoring systems. The area required for each bed would be the same as a general ward, but each bed space requires oxygen, suction and electrical outlets. Ideally the unit should be close to others dealing with acutely ill patients.

Operational policies need to be clearly defined. Each unit must have agreed admission and discharge policies. A clinical co-ordinator would be of value, not in clinical management, but to ensure communication and correct observation of guidelines. He/she could also hold the unit's budget.

Formal rotations and training programmes will be necessary for medical and nursing staff to maintain expertise.

Report of the Joint Working Party on Graduated Patient Care

Guidelines on efficient provision of services for patients with different levels of clinical dependency.

SUMMARY

Graduated patient care is a concept which allows stratification of patients according to clinical dependency into those who:

- *should be admitted to an intensive care unit (ICU) for the management of single or multiple organ failure*
- *should best be treated in a high dependency unit (HDU)*
- *can be adequately treated on a general surgical ward*
- *are clinically stable and self-caring and can be managed on a convalescent unit or hotel unit*
- *have a long-term disability and require care in a long stay unit.*

Good clinical practice requires that special skills and expensive equipment are concentrated where they are most needed, and where the available skills and technology can be used to the best advantage.

- *Patients who need artificial ventilation or management of single or multiple organ failure need the specialised facility and dedicated nursing available on an intensive care unit. Surveys indicate that about 5–10% of surgical patients need considerably more care than is generally available in standard surgical wards linked to the availability of continuous monitoring. High dependency units should be provided in district general hospitals as an intermediate step between intensive care and general ward care.*
- *Analysis of the re-organisation of services in a district general hospital indicates that overall nursing staff requirements should remain neutral, but an operational study under the auspices of the multidisciplinary team, and including measurements of the quality of care, is needed.*
- *The variable demands posed by emergency and seriously ill patients create difficulties in most hospitals, and an architectural study demonstrates how this problem can be eased by providing flexibility in bed space planning.*

Published in January 1996 by The Royal College of Anaesthetists and The Royal College of Surgeons of England and reproduced with permission from The Royal College of Surgeons of England.

The Role of the Anaesthetist in the Emergency Services

Standards for the provision in Accident and Emergency departments of anaesthesia, resuscitation, major incident management and other services involving anaesthetists.

ANAESTHESIA AND ANALGESIA IN A&E

The standard of anaesthetic care and safety must be the same as in any other area.

Location/equipment
Appropriate anaesthetic monitoring, and resuscitation equipment, as well as an appropriately staffed area for recovery, must be provided. A nominated consultant anaesthetist should be responsible for these facilities.

Personnel
All consultant anaesthetists should be familiar with the facilities in A&E. A trained anaesthetic nurse or ODA should be present whenever anaesthesia is conducted.

Patient selection
Most patients will be ASA I or II. Patients who are ASA II or IV may be acceptable for short, minor procedures. The anaesthetist must be satisfied with post discharge arrangements where the patient is not admitted to hospital.

Precautions against aspiration of gastric contents are advisable up to 12 hours after trauma.

Children require special facilities, and the needs of parents should be considered.

Local anaesthetic infiltration and peripheral nerve blocks
These are safe, provided non-toxic doses are used and there are no contraindications. If safety measures are adopted, a single operator/anaesthetist is acceptable, provided he/she is trained in basic resuscitation.

Intravenous regional anaesthesia and major regional analgesia
These can be hazardous. One person should carry out the procedure while another person with advanced life support skills looks after the patient. Intravenous regional anaesthesia (IVRA) should only be used by a person skilled and experienced in its use. IVRA equipment should be maintained regularly and checked before use.

Published in July 1991 by The Association of Anaesthetists of Great Britain and Ireland.

Sedation
Sedation should only be administered by those with suitable training and experience. Overdose is a risk in frail elderly patients, but also in young patients who become restless. Supplementary oxygen and pulse oximetry are strongly recommended.

Recovery and discharge
Recovery facilities and discharge arrangements should be comparable with those in day case units. The patient should be assessed for 'street fitness'. Specific written instructions should be given in relation to driving, etc.

RESUSCITATION IN THE A&E DEPARTMENT

Arrangements for a resuscitation service should be made by the nominated consultant anaesthetist in co-operation with the consultant in charge of the A&E department.

Arrangements should ensure 24 hour skilled anaesthetic cover, adequate equipment for resuscitation, adequate patient monitoring equipment, satisfactory arrangements for patient transfer within and between hospitals and a regular schedule of maintenance of all equipment.

Training
All staff should receive basic life support training, medical staff should receive advanced life support training, anaesthetic and A&E medical staff should receive advanced trauma life support training.

Audit
An audit of anaesthetic and resuscitation services in A&E should be carried out. Audit may be facilitated by the use of scoring system, such as the TRISS method.

MAJOR INCIDENTS

Major incident plans
The nominated consultant anaesthetist should be a member of the hospital's major incident committee. Plans need to take account of potential local incidents in industry, airports, etc., and should be reviewed regularly.

Clinical responsibilities
The anaesthetic department provides a number of services, including membership of the on-site team, triage and pain relief, resuscitation in A&E, co-ordination and provision of anaesthetic services for people requiring surgery, intensive care or high dependency care.

Call out
Call out should be by a prearranged plan, using a 'telephone cascade'. Action cards should be issued to all personnel likely to be called. Photo-i.d. cards permit identification of staff by security staff or police.

On-site role

Triage, resuscitation, pain relief and occasionally anaesthesia will be required at the site of an incident.

Mobile teams consist of four people: an experienced anaesthetist, a surgeon or A&E doctor and two nurses or ODAs. They should normally be sent to the site from a hospital which is not the major designated receiving hospital. A Medical Incident Officer should be brought to the site as soon as possible. His/her role is to supervise and liaise.

Protective clothing, with identifying marks, must be worn. Portable first aid and resuscitation equipment should be carried in weatherproof containers.

All members of the team should be covered by adequate insurance. Cover provided by the DoH is often inadequate and trusts should arrange additional cover.

Communications

All communications between site and hospital should principally be via a radio link with the ambulance service. On-site team leaders should have two-way radio. Mobile phones can be useful early on, but batteries wear down, and the cell net rapidly becomes saturated.

Training

Training includes ATLS and ALS courses and clinical practice gained at, for example, dangerous sporting events. It also includes exercises, post-event audit and counselling.

TRAINING OF AMBULANCE AND PARAMEDICAL STAFF

At least 60% of emergency ambulance crew members should be trained to paramedic standards.

Curriculum

Extended training of ambulance personnel is the responsibility of the NHS Training Authority Special Projects Group, which has an anaesthetist as a member. Anaesthetists have a particular contribution to make to training in airway management, ventilation and circulatory support. Training will also cover assessment and control of blood loss, intravenous access and infusions, ECG interpretation and the use of certain drugs.

Consent and responsibility

Anaesthetists should ensure that their employer has agreed to extend their vicarious liability in respect of training ambulance staff, and that trainee ambulance staff are covered by their employers. Training of any kind requires patient consent.

DUTIES, COMMITMENT AND SUPPORT

The consultant(s) co-ordinating anaesthetic services in A&E is responsible for:

- liaison with A&E staff, and other members of the anaesthetic department
- direction of anaesthetic services inside and outside the hospital
- involvement with major incident plans
- a commitment to training paramedics and other staff.

His/her job plan should have an allowance of one NHD for up to 25 000 patients per year treated in A&E and *pro rata* for busier departments. Anaesthetists heavily involved with paramedic training should negotiate an appropriate NHD allowance

There should be secretarial support and an adequate budget for equipment and training.

NHS Management Changes: Implications for Anaesthetists

The advice of the Association on implications of the Health Service reforms to anaesthetists.

INTRODUCTION

The Council stresses three over-riding messages.

- *Do not throw away one of the specialty's greatest strengths – the unity of working groups of colleagues who stick by jointly agreed local policies which are in the majority interest.*
- *Do adhere to the national guidelines which have been prepared over successive years by The Association of Anaesthetists of Great Britain and Ireland and by The Royal College of Anaesthetists. They have provided extremely good quality control over the standards of anaesthetists.*
- *Do not leave management to the managers. Clinical directors in particular and clinicians in general have a golden opportunity to work in conjunction with managers to bring substantial improvements in hospital management and to patient care. The opportunity must not be wasted.*

BUSINESS PLANS

Clinical directorates
These are the principal system of management for hospital resources. Departments of anaesthesia should seek their own separate clinical directorate. These directorates should be able to identify costs and resources needed to provide services, which requires the creation of a business plan. Quality of service should be an important part of such a business plan.

Business planning
Business planning for an anaesthetic directorate will define the current service and its cost, plan for future changes and establish ways to maintain and develop quality. The plan will have to demonstrate awareness of the policies and plans of the purchasers, and other clinical directorates.

An outline business plan is as follows.

1. Mission statement.
2. Aims and objectives.
3. Service capacity: organisation and management, staffing, facilities, allocation of time.

Published in September 1992 by The Association of Anaesthetists of Great Britain and Ireland. The Introduction is reproduced with permission from The Association of Anaesthetists of Great Britain and Ireland.

4. Utilisation: number of cases, emergency component, ICU services, obstetric services, acute and non-acute pain services, available resuscitation and A&E services, teaching responsibilities, any areas of special interest (cardiac, neuro, etc.).
5. Financial resources.
6. SWOT analysis (= Strengths, Weaknesses, Opportunities, Threats).
7. Objectives for the coming year: meeting deficiencies, improving efficiency, areas of development and their cost implications.

Quality of service

This has cost implications, but the hospital will suffer in the long term where quality is not high. Quality also includes education of trainees, and consultants should be encouraged to participate in regional and professional activities to maintain standards, and keep accreditation by the College. The Clinical Director should ensure the provision of educational programmes, funded study leave, and the development of an effective audit system.

ANAESTHETIC BUDGETS AND CONTRACTS

Purchasers and providers

Anaesthetists work in provider units. Purchasers include the local district Health Authority, GP fundholders, other Health Authorities and private patients or their agents.

Anaesthetic budget management arrangements

These may be set up in various ways.

1. The Clinical Director responsible for providing the services may hold the budget for all anaesthetic services (including ICU, pain, etc.). **This is the arrangement favoured by the Association**.
2. The budget for anaesthetic services may be held within other directorates.
3. The department of anaesthesia may hold a budget just for medical staff and secretaries, budgets for theatre and ICU staff being held elsewhere.
4. In some hospitals, there are no clinical directors, and budgets are only devolved as far as non-clinical general managers.

GP fundholders

GP fundholders only hold budgets for elective services at present, including outpatient referrals, elective surgery, diagnostic services and domicillary visits. They play an important part in the purchasing of anaesthetic services.

GP fundholders are concerned with cost and quality of services. Throughput, length of stay and complication rates affect these variables. The value of those 'anaesthetic services' which improve quality of care without affecting throughput or length of stay should be made known to all purchasers.

Purchasing contracts

These contracts come in three types.

1. Block contracts provide a sum of money to cover all patient referrals in a given year, regardless of number.
2. Cost and volume contracts imply that additional payments at marginal cost can be made if the work exceeds the contracted volume or, in some cases, reductions in funding made if the contracted volume is not achieved.
3. Cost per case is a price for each item of work undertaken. Many hospitals do not yet have reliable data to produce such a price.

Actual prices exist for all services in each hospital, and anaesthetists should have access to them.

Budget income
This is determined by the Management Board and makes assumptions regarding contract income (based on block or cost and volume income) and other income (from cost per case purchasing and extra-contractual referrals). The anaesthetic budget should receive its share of any unplanned income from the latter source.

Budget setting
This takes place annually and involves the clinical director, nurse manager, business manager and the hospital finance department. It begins by identifying and tackling any potential shortfall in funding existing services, before setting the budget for the following year.

Conclusion
The changes to the NHS are not just cosmetic. The future budget of the directorate depends on securing contracts and accurately predicting the real price of the service. Anaesthetists who do not involve themselves in this activity risk inadequate funding and reduced job satisfaction.

COSTING OF ANAESTHETIC SERVICES

Elements of service cost
1. Staff costs: medical, nursing, managerial, technical, administrative, ancillary. The budget should include the full gross salary cost, including national insurance and superannuation. It should include a provision for recruitment costs.
2. Equipment: the asset register, where it exists, should identify the equipment available. Costing should include full servicing costs (approximately 10% of capital costs per annum on average). NHS rules allow for an annual capital charge to be debited to the Directorate's budget for depreciation, and a notional interest charge of 6%. Capital charges assume a life of 10 years for mechanical equipment and 5 years for electronic equipment and ventilators.
3. Consumables and drugs receive much attention despite representing a small part of overall cost.

Costing methods
1. Personal billing apportions specific costs to individual patients.
2. A case mix approach takes the total annual cost and apportions it either *per capita*, or *per capita* per hour.

3. Average costs are calculated by dividing the costs of anaesthetic room items by the number of cases. The figure can then be applied to a range of procedures.
4. A simpler alternative is to cost the consumables being delivered to anaesthetic rooms. This approach can lead to items being costed to anaesthesia when used by others, for example intravenous antibiotics.

Additional costing issues
*   Vacancy factor: some hospitals reduce the staffing budget by as much as 5% to allow for turnover vacancies.
*   Special high cost services such as intensive care costs need to be taken into account.
*   Recharging mechanisms, where one directorate charges another for the use of anaesthetic services, may develop in the future.
*   Marginal costs, that is the cost incurred by one extra unit of service, are always less than average cost, and must be calculated accurately for cost and volume contracts.

Hospital overheads
These include capital and service charges for the hospital site, and must be considered when determining the final price of services. Where there is pressure for efficiency savings, this should be applied equally to hospital overheads and to directorates.

TERMS AND CONDITIONS OF SERVICE

Consultant appointments
Trust hospitals are not bound by national terms and conditions.

Local Negotiating Committees are considered essential when negotiating with trusts. Trusts which ignore British Medical Association (BMA) requirements are likely to have problems with recruitment.

Present post holders may possibly be offered alterations in contract, but must be aware of the implications of accepting alternatives to nationally agreed packages.

New appointees may not be offered NHS contracts, and must be aware of the implications of accepting limited term contracts. BMA Industrial Relations Officers can offer advice.

NHS terms and conditions may not continue to exist long into the future. Given the shortage of anaesthetists, trusts may put pressure on anaesthetists to undertake more NHDs than are recommended. Where additional payments are made for extra work, they are paid at basic rate and are not superannuable.

Non-consultant career grades should be used in a manner appropriate to their training and to service need. Creation of new non-consultant career grades should be discouraged.

Training implications
The position of trainees is protected to some degree, given that their contracts will not be altered unfavourably. Trainees should not be pressed into additional commitment by their employer or senior colleagues.

Extra-contractual work

Waiting list initiative (WLI) work undertaken in NHS hospitals is covered by Crown Indemnity. Wherever it is conducted, payment for such work is included within the 10% maximum for private practice earnings, and is not superannuable.

Association advice

The Association advises that contracts should be negotiated as a department or directorate.

The Patient's Charter

A selection of the rights and standards pertinent to anaesthesia contained in the document 'The Patient's Charter and You'.

- You have the right to receive health care on the basis of your clinical need, not on your ability to pay, lifestyle or any other factor.
- You have the right to get emergency treatment at any time through your GP, the emergency ambulance service and hospital A&E departments.
- You have the right to choose whether or not you want to take part in medical research or medical student training.
- You can expect all the staff you meet face to face to wear name badges.
- You can expect the NHS to respect your privacy, dignity and religious and cultural beliefs at all times and in all places. For example, meals should suit your dietary and religious needs. Staff should ask you whether you want to be called by your first or last name and respect your preference.
- You have the right to have any proposed treatment, including any risks involved in that treatment and any alternatives, clearly explained to you before you decide whether to agree to it. You have the right to have access to your health records, and to know that everyone working for the NHS is under legal duty to keep your records confidential.
- For hip or knee replacements and cataract operations, a waiting time guarantee of 18 months has already been established.
- From April 1995, the NHS is broadening this 18-month guarantee to cover all admissions to hospital.
- In addition, from April 1995, you can expect treatment within 1 year for coronary artery bypass grafts and some associated procedures. (If your consultant considers your need for treatment is urgent, you can expect to be seen much more quickly than this.)
- Your operation should not be cancelled on the day you are due to go into hospital or after you have gone in. If it is (for example, because the hospital is dealing with the victims of a major road accident), you can expect to be admitted again within 1 month of the cancellation.
- If you go to an A&E department, you can expect to be seen immediately and have your need for treatment assessed.
- From April 1996, if you are admitted to hospital through an A&E department, you can expect to be given a bed as soon as possible, and certainly within 2 hours.
- If you agree, you can expect your relatives and friends to be kept up to date with the progress of your treatment.

Published in November 1996 by the Department of Health.

The Report of the Confidential Enquiry into Perioperative Deaths

CONCLUSIONS

1. The overall death rate after anaesthesia and surgery, analysed in this enquiry, was low. The mortality in over half a million operations was 0.7% and most of these deaths were in the elderly (over 75 years old) and were unavoidable due to progression of the presenting condition, such as advanced cancer, or co-existing diseases such as heart and/or respiratory failure. Death was solely attributable to avoidable surgical or anaesthetic factors in a very small proportion of patients.
2. The majority of clinicians in the relevant disciplines co-operated in this system of clinical audit.
3. There were important differences in clinical practice between the three regions studied.
4. There were also deficiencies in the Hospital Activity Analysis data. There were also problems with the storage, movement and retrieval of patients' notes, particularly those of deceased patients.
5. Many surgeons and anaesthetists did not hold regular audits of their operation results (mortality and morbidity meetings). The proportion varied with the sub-specialty, but joint meetings between the two disciplines were very rare.
6. There were important differences in the consultants' supervision of trainees.
7. There were a number of deaths in which junior surgeons or anaesthetists did not seek the advice of their consultants or senior registrars at any time before, during or after the operations.
8. The preoperative assessment and resuscitation of patients by doctors of both disciplines was sometimes compromised by undue haste to operate. This was a greater problem than delayed operations, and it is possible that pressure to fit an operation into a very tight theatre schedule was one of the factors responsible.
9. There were instances of patients who were moribund or terminally ill having operations that would not have improved their condition.
10. There were examples of surgeons operating for conditions for which they were not trained, or performing operations outside their field of primary expertise.
11. There were examples of difficulties in transferring patients for specialised treatment to other hospitals in the area.

RECOMMENDATIONS

Quality assurance
* *There is a need for an assessment of clinical practice on a national basis. Our experience suggests that our colleagues would welcome this.*
* *Consultants in every district should ensure that their own coding and input to information systems (including the Körner systems) is accurate and up-to-date; without this any audit is flawed. Every district should urgently review the storage, movement, and retrieval of patients' notes, particularly those of deceased patients.*

Published in 1987 by The National Confidential Enquiry into Perioperative Deaths and reproduced with their permission.

- *Clinicians need to assess themselves regularly. Effective self-assessment needs time; time to attend autopsies, mortality/morbidity meetings and clinical review with other disciplines.*

Accountability

All departments of anaesthetics and surgery should review their arrangements for consultants' supervision of trainees. Locally agreed guidelines are important to ensure appropriate care of all patients, but particularly when responsibility is transferred from one clinical team, or shift, to another. No senior house officer or registrar should undertake any anaesthetic or surgical operation as an emergency or urgent matter without consultation with their consultant (or senior registrar).

Clinical decision making

- *Resuscitation, assessment and management of medical disease take time and may determine outcome; their importance needs to be re-stated. Arrangements which permit this in everycase are important.*
- *The decision to operate on the elderly and very sick is important and should be taken at consultant (or senior registrar) level. For the most seriously ill patients, consultant anaesthetists and surgeons should consult together before the operation.*
- *The decision **not** to operate is difficult. Humanity suggests that patients who are terminally ill should not have operations (i.e. non-life-saving), but should be allowed to die in peace with dignity.*

Organisational issues

- *Districts should review their facilities for out of hours work and concentrate anaesthetic surgical and nursing resources at a single location. A fully staffed and fully equipped anaesthetic room, resuscitation room, operating room, recovery area and high dependency or intensive therapy unit should be available at all times.*
- *The implementation of the CEPOD classification of operations (emergency, urgent, scheduled and elective) would concentrate the attention of all staff on the fact that very few operations need to be performed at night.*
- *Operations should only be performed by consultants or junior surgeons (accountable to consultants) who have had adequate training in the specialty relevant to that operation. Health Authorities should therefore balance surgical specialties so that appropriate urological and vascular trained surgeons are provided in each district. In the case of small districts this may necessitate sub-Regional units to ensure adequate sub-speciality care. Neurological and neonatal surgery should be carried out at special regional units.*

The Report of the National Confidential Enquiry into Perioperative Deaths 1989

RECOMMENDATIONS

1. *The National Confidential Enquiry into Perioperative Deaths should continue.*
2. *The information systems, particularly clinical information systems, in the NHS should be considerably improved to provide accurate and timely information for audit and clinical quality assurance. All consultants should assist in achieving this improvement.*
3. *Local audit meetings are essential to good clinical practice, and all consultants should participate.*
4. *Surgeons and anaesthetists should not undertake occasional paediatric practice. The outcome of surgery and anaesthesia in children is related to the experience of the clinicians involved.*
5. *Consultants who take responsibility for the care of children (particularly in district general hospitals) must keep up to date and competent in the management of children.*
6. *Consultant supervision of trainees needs to be kept under scrutiny. No trainee should undertake any anaesthetic or surgical operation on a child of any age without consultation with their consultant.*

Published in June 1990 by The National Confidential Enquiry into Perioperative Deaths and reproduced with their permission.

The Report of the National Confidential Enquiry into Perioperative Deaths 1990

The National Confidential Enquiry into Perioperative Deaths is concerned with the quality of the delivery of anaesthesia and surgery: it does not study the causation of death. Many of the patients mentioned in the report were old, very seriously ill and were expected to die by the doctors who cared for them. The report contains recommendations about improvements in the care of patients. There are no **new** lessons.

GENERAL CONCLUSIONS

*The conclusions are relevant to both the **medical profession** and to **managers**.*

1. *Information. There are examples throughout the report about deficiencies in the hospital notes; at least 90 cases could not be studied because notes were acknowledged to be lost. Operation notes were sometimes missing or lacking in essential details such as the name of the surgeon or the diagnosis; anaesthetic notes regularly failed to record physiological changes. Hospital notes about dead patients tend to given a low priority by records staff and soon disappear and become difficult to read.*
2. *Essential services. Recovery rooms, high dependency units and intensive care units need not merely exist as structures, they must also be ready for use. Proper equipment and qualified specialist staff (nurses, operating department assistants) must be available at all times if patients are to survive anaesthesia and surgery. If these services are not available patients may have to moved elsewhere. Services were noted to be deficient, or closed on Bank Holidays (particularly Christmas) and, perhaps surprisingly at night. The proper and safe provision of pain relief after surgery implies that more high dependency units are required.*
3. *Emergency operating rooms. The provision of this essential service is important for all surgical specialities. Best results are obtained when there is no (non-medical) delay in the management of, for example, fractured neck of femur. If patients are to receive the greatest benefit from modern surgery it must be performed at the clinically most opportune moment. Dedicated operating rooms for emergency surgery are an essential service for all surgical specialities.*
4. *Split sites. The problems caused by the requirement for Consultants and their teams) to work and be on call regularly on more than one NHS site are well known. The use of split sites should be historical.*
5. *Consultants. In this Enquiry, 83% of the decisions about surgery were made by Consultants or Senior Registrars.*
6. *About half the anaesthetics for the group of patients who subsequently died were conducted in the precise knowledge and (or) presence of a Consultant. This proportion is not yet satisfactory but many of the deaths occurred as a result of factors outside the clinical responsibility of anaesthetists.*
7. *Speciality involvement. A few surgeons persist in occasional operating outside their primary speciality; this is deplored.*
8. *Locums. Temporary appointments are sometimes necessary. The most senior operating surgeon was a locum in 7% of the deaths; similarly, 9% of anaesthetists **working alone** were*

Published in April 1992 by The National Confidential Enquiry into Perioperative Deaths and reproduced with their permission.

locums. Sometimes these locums, of both disciplines, were 'acting up' but too often they admitted personally that they were inadequately trained or out of practice at particular procedures.

9. *Non-medical assistance.* The need for trained non-medically qualified assistants for anaesthetists is overwhelming; in 59% of deaths the anaesthetist was working without medical assistance.

10. *Post mortem examinations.* The infrequency of this useful investigation revealed in this Enquiry is to be deplored. Communication between pathologists (both hospital and Coroners') and clinicians is so poor that useful lessons can often not be learnt.

11. *Non-trainee, non-Consultant clinicians.* There is evidence within this report that these clinicians (Associate Specialist, Staff Grade, Clinical Assistant) are sometimes isolated. Arrangements whereby these individuals are fully integrated into departments of surgery and anaesthesia need to be improved. This should include involvement in audit meetings.

12. *Supervision.* Trainee surgeons and anaesthetists need to be encouraged to request supervision. Consultants must ensure that trainees have the confidence to ask and to know that their request will not be rebuffed. If proper supervision of trainees is to be achieved, there may need to be more Consultants, particularly in orthopaedic surgery and anaesthesia.

13. *Confidential enquiries.* The influence of confidential enquiries in the practice of medicine in the United Kingdom is undeniable. The effects of CEPOD and NCEPOD are such that this unique enquiry should continue.

GENERAL RECOMMENDATIONS

1. *The provision of clinical and management information about patients, including post mortem records, needs to improved significantly.*

2. *Essential services (including staffed emergency rooms, recovery rooms, high dependency units and intensive care units) must be provided on a single site wherever emergency/acute surgical care is delivered.*

3. *Decisions for or against operations should be made jointly by surgeons and anaesthetists; this is a Consultant responsibility.*

4. *The supervision of locum appointments at all grades in anaesthesia and surgery needs urgent review.*

5. *All grades of surgeon and anaesthetist should be involved in medical audit and continuing medical education.*

6. *Efforts should be made to increase the number of post mortem examinations.*

7. *The National Confidential Enquiry into Perioperative Deaths should continue.*

The Report of the National Confidential Enquiry into Perioperative Deaths 1991/1992

GENERAL RECOMMENDATIONS

- *The medical Royal Colleges and the Specialist Societies in Surgery, Gynaecology and Anaesthesia must encourage all Consultants to participate in The National Confidential Enquiry into Perioperative Deaths. Full co-operation would enable the profession to defend itself against charges of falling standards and lack of public accountability. The failure of some Consultants to return questionnaires is unacceptable and a cause for concern.*
- *Surgeons, gynaecologists and anaesthetists need to address the continuing problem of thromboembolism which causes death after surgery. We have emphasised this matter before and we regret that we must again bring the profession's attention to it. Hospitals and clinical directorates should be required to address the issue and develop an agreed protocol. Every Consultant should then follow this protocol. The research bodies and the Department of Health need to continue actively to encourage and support research in this field.*
- *All grades of surgeons, gynaecologists and anaesthetists must realise the critical importance of fluid balance in elderly patients.*
- *There needs to be a collaborative approach to the matching of surgical and anaesthetic skills to the condition of the patient.*
- *Surgeons, gynaecologists and anaesthetists must have immediate access to essential services (recovery rooms, high dependency and intensive care units) if their patients are to survive. The previous Reports have emphasised the need to have emergency operating and recovery rooms available 24 hours a day.*
- *It is no longer acceptable for basic specialist trainees (Senior House Officers) in some specialities to work alone without suitable supervision and direction by their Consultant. Managers and Consultants must locally achieve these arrangements.*
- *The post mortem rate is too low. At least 49% of post mortems demonstrate, despite clinicians' scepticism, significant, new and unexpected findings which are relevant. Post mortems are an important form of quality control.*

The necessary information available within the NHS under the present system is inadequate. Despite our repeated comment about this, we are still unable to obtain basic and timely data about the number of patients who have operations and the number of perioperative deaths. There is a need for an improved method for collection and validation of information on perioperative deaths locally and nationally.

IMPORTANT ISSUES IN MANAGEMENT

- *Managers must realise that there are resource implications for a service which is increasingly Consultant-based.*
- *Managers should urgently review the storage and retrieval of medical notes.*
- *Managers should assist local reporters to identify methods of reporting **all** relevant deaths.*
- *Data on the number of surgical procedures performed and the number of perioperative deaths will be inadequate until a unique patient number is in general use in all medical records.*

Published in September 1993 by The National Confidential Enquiry into Perioperative Deaths and reproduced with their permission.

IMPORTANT ISSUES IN SURGERY

- *Surgery should be avoided for those whose death is inevitable and imminent. A more humane approach to the care of these patients should be considered; these decisions should be directed by Consultants.*
- *Specialist opinion should be sought before undertaking some procedures (for example, amputation, oesophagectomy, hysterectomy, craniotomy).*
- *Resuscitation and preparation of patients for surgery should not be inadequate or hasty (for example, strangulated hernia).*
- *There is a need for more consultant involvement in the theatre, particularly for emergency cases (for example, colorectal resection).*

IMPORTANT ISSUES IN ANAESTHESIA

- *Arrangements whereby anaesthetists could work in teams (with other anaesthetists) should be considered.*
- *Anaesthetists should review their practice of non-invasive instrumental monitoring at induction of anaesthesia.*
- *The potential for local protocols or national guidelines for staff–patient matching, the use of anaesthesia teams, the provision of essential services, the transfer of patients and other matters should be realised.*

The Report of the National Confidential Enquiry into Perioperative Deaths 1992/1993

GENERAL RECOMMENDATIONS

- *NCEPOD has again identified the substantial shortfall in critical care services. Any hospital admitting emergency patients, and hospitals admitting complex elective patients, must have adequate facilities for intensive and/or high dependency care at all times.*
- *Trainees with less than 3 years' training in the specialty should not anaesthetise or operate without appropriate supervision.*
- *Practitioners must recognise their own limitations and not hesitate to consult a more appropriate colleague when managing conditions outside their immediate expertise.*
- *The skills of the surgeon and anaesthetist should always be appropriate for the physiological and pathological state of the patient.*
- *Surgeons operating laparoscopically should not hesitate to convert to an open approach when necessary.*
- *Appropriately trained staff must accompany all patients with life-threatening conditions during transfer between and within hospitals.*
- *The medical profession needs to develop and enforce standards of practice for the management of many common acute conditions (e.g. head injuries, aortic aneurysm, colorectal cancer, gastrointestinal bleeding).*
- *There is an urgent need to improve the quality of medical notes.*
- *Managers need to improve the services provided by medical records departments so that notes are available when requested.*

Published in November 1995 by The National Confidential Enquiry into Perioperative Deaths and reproduced with their permission.

The Report of the National Confidential Enquiry into Perioperative Deaths 1993/1994

GENERAL RECOMMENDATIONS

- *Consultation, collaboration and teamwork between anaesthetists surgeons and physicians should be encouraged and should be the usual practice.*
- *Surgical management should be planned and should include all those provisions that are required for good outcomes.*
- *The availability of staffed (medical, nursing and ancillary) emergency operating theatres on a 24-hour basis is essential; Trusts admitting urgent and emergency cases must ensure they are provided.*
- *The elderly and unfit constitute a large proportion of the workload; improved perioperative management is required to ensure that their care is appropriate.*
- *Protocols for the treatment of common conditions should be applied more widely to both elective and emergency admissions, and should be subject to audit.*
- *Continuity of care after operations is essential; local arrangements must ensure that it occurs.*
- *The roles and responsibilities of all doctors need to be more clearly defined nationally, and implemented locally.*
- *Clinicians and Coroners should make strenuous efforts to improve their local working relationships.*
- *Systems should be implemented by trusts to improve the retention and availability of all notes and records of clinical activity.*
- *Trusts need to encourage more participation in clinical audit.*
- *More research is required on thromboembolism prophylaxis.*

Published in November 1996 by The National Confidential Enquiry into Perioperative Deaths and reproduced with their permission.

National ITU Audit 1992/1993

This audit was based on a questionnaire survey of all units in the UK believed to have an intensive care unit. A total of 277 questionnaires were sent and 256 were completed (92%).

CONCLUSIONS

1. Many ITUs are very small, and may admit small numbers of patients, many of which could be cared for in an HDU. Many of them function with inadequate numbers of staff, and may have to refuse admissions or transfer patients.
2. In almost half the units, medical records are inadequate for the purposes of outcome measurement.
3. The fact that many units still provide a high level of service under such circumstances can only be due to dedication and overwork on a large scale.
4. Less than 40% of units have enough consultant medical time to provide 24-hour cover. The fact that 15 units have no allocated consultant sessions is unacceptable.
5. Eighty five units either had no resident or failed to reply to the relevant question. Even if only half of these have no resident, it is unacceptable.
6. If the present circumstances are allowed to continue, trainees passing through ITUs will have little or no training.
7. Those trainees who intend to pursue a career in which intensive therapy will play a major role must undergo a period of structured training recognised by the Royal Colleges.
8. Only 34 units admitted more than 21 children in the year under review. It is not possible to arrive at a figure for paediatric admissions which would guarantee the appropriate skills acquisition and maintenance.
9. The diffusion of ITU patients into small units cannot provide high quality training opportunities. Patients are being transferred between units, and in some areas it has become routine.
10. Regionalisation of intensive therapy services is recommended to improve patient care, training and efficient use of resources.

Published in 1993 by The Royal College of Anaesthetists.

Report on Confidential Enquiries into Maternal Deaths in the United Kingdom 1985–87

- Six early deaths and two late deaths were directly attributable to anaesthesia in this triennium.
- Anaesthesia contributed to death in a further 16 women: five associated with cardiac disease, four with haemorrhage, three with hypertensive disorders and four with miscellaneous problems.
- Tracheal tube problems and failure of organisation and postoperative care were common. Monitoring was often inadequate.

DIRECT ANAESTHETIC DEATHS

Difficulty with tracheal intubation (four deaths)

1. Elective Caesarean section for cephalopelvic disproportion. Offered epidural but chose general anaesthesia. Failure to detect oesophageal intubation led to death from cerebral anoxia.
2. Planned emergency Caesarean section for failure to progress. Epidural placed for labour which worked well, but despite top-ups could not produce adequate anaesthesia for Caesarean section. Given general anaesthesia, vocal cords not visualised but intubation was thought to have been achieved. The patient was given 20 mg of alcuronium, but hypoxia developed and the tube was removed. The patient was manually ventilated with a face mask. Death occurred 2 days later in the ICU as a result of the hypoxic episode. The anaesthetist had no skilled assistance.
3. Grossly obese patient underwent emergency Caesarean section for fetal distress. She had proteinuria, oedema and hypertension. Intubation was difficult but the tube was thought to be in the trachea. Breath sounds were audible. Non-depolarising muscle relaxants were given. The patient suffered severe hypoxia and a cardiac arrest. Despite attempts at a tracheostomy, the patient could not be resuscitated.
4. A woman was admitted in labour with a concealed pregnancy, blood pressure 110 mmHg diastolic. She delivered a stillborn infant. She was given general anaesthesia for removal of a retained placenta. The patient failed to breathe after surgery, and suxamethonium apnoea was suspected. She was transferred to an HDU for ventilation, but suffered hypoxia as a result of a kinked tracheal tube, and died.

Late deaths

- A woman who underwent emergency Caesarean section under general anaesthesia for fetal distress suffered hypoxia and severe brain damage as a result of an undetected oesophageal intubation. She died after many months without regaining consciousness.
- A woman, known to have been difficult to intubate at previous Caesarean section, received general anaesthesia for an elective Caesarean section. Intubation was not possible and the patient was woken up. An epidural was sited, but when 8 ml of 0.5% bupivacaine was given, the patient rapidly became hypotensive and stopped breathing. During resuscitation, oesophageal intubation occurred which was not detected for some time. The patient suffered severe brain damage and subsequently died.

Published in 1991 by HMSO.

Comment: It is important to ensure that the patient is adequately anaesthetised prior to intubation; there must be a full range of equipment; skilled assistance should be provided; cricoid pressure is a two-handed technique; a failed intubation drill should be agreed and practised by all those involved in obstetric anaesthesia.

Aspiration of gastric contents (one death)
The patient received general anaesthesia for Caesarean section, and despite the use of an accepted method of antacid prophylaxis (ranitidine and sodium citrate), and cricoid pressure, aspiration occurred at induction, which subsequently led to her death.

Cardiac disease (one death)
The patient had aortic incompetence, complicated by heart failure and pre-eclampsia. She underwent Caesarean section at 32 weeks because of increasing cardiac failure. An epidural was sited. A test dose of 2 ml of 0.5% bupivacaine was followed by a single dose of 18 ml of 0.5% bupivacaine, followed by a further injection of 6 ml of 0.5% bupivacaine. Profound cardiovascular collapse occurred, and resuscitation was unsuccessful.

Comment: the choice of anaesthetic in patients with cardiac failure is controversial; invasive monitoring is essential; fractionating the dose of local anaesthetic may have helped; general anaesthesia may have caused less hypotension.

Report on Confidential Enquiries into Maternal Deaths in the United Kingdom 1988–90

- There were 15 deaths associated with anaesthesia in this triennium; four directly due to anaesthesia, one late death directly due to anaesthesia and 10 cases in which anaesthesia was thought to have contributed to death.
- Of the direct anaesthetic deaths, one was the result of a tracheal tube problem, one of pulmonary oedema after spinal anaesthesia, one of substandard postoperative care and two (including the late death) were caused by aspiration of gastric contents.

DIRECT ANAESTHETIC DEATHS

Tracheal tube obstruction

A patient underwent emergency planned Caesarean section for pre-eclampsia and fetal distress. The anaesthetist (an SHO with 10 months' experience) attempted a spinal, but subsequently abandoned the technique in favour of general anaesthesia, during which the patient could not be intubated. Failed intubation procedure was followed, and a consultant anaesthetist was summoned who was able to intubate the trachea. Shortly after delivery of the baby, airway pressure increased, severe hypoxia developed and, despite repositioning the tube, cardiac arrest occurred. The tube cuff was deflated and the tube moved down the trachea and back again. This resulted in normal inflation pressures and cardiac rhythm. The patient suffered diffuse brain damage and was transferred to the ICU. Some weeks later the patient died during tracheostomy under general anaesthesia, in association with difficulty in ventilation through the tracheostomy tube.

Pulmonary oedema after spinal anaesthesia

An obese woman was admitted at 30 weeks for drainage and marsupialisation of a Bartholin's abscess. The patient agreed to a spinal anaesthetic. After a preload of 400 ml of Hartmann's solution, 1.0 ml of 0.5% heavy bupivacaine was injected in the sitting position. After 1 minute, the patient noticed weakness in the legs. Eight minutes after injection, blood pressure dropped to 75/28 mmHg. Treatment with 600 ml of Hartmann's, two doses of 15 mg intravenous ephedrine, 600 ml of synthetic colloid, failed to increase the blood pressure, and at this point the pulse dropped to 40–50/min. Oxygen and three doses of 0.6 mg atropine were given, with no effect on the blood pressure. One ml of 1:1000 adrenaline was given, which restored blood pressure to 135/86 mmHg, and pulse to 104/min. Within 20 minutes, the patient started to cough up pink frothy sputum, and became tachypnoeic, hypoxaemic and hypotensive. The patient was intubated and transferred to the intensive care unit where she died 11 days later of adult respiratory distress syndrome (ARDS).

Inadequate postoperative care

The patient was very obese, a heavy smoker and a chronic hypertensive treated with atenolol. During a prolonged first stage, she received epidural analgesia. After 8 hours

Published in 1994 by HMSO.

she underwent Caesarean section under general anaesthesia, having refused to have the operation under epidural alone. The operation was uneventful. Fifteen minutes after extubation, breathing became laboured, and blood pressure dropped to 70/30 mmHg. The anaesthetist was called, gave an intravenous dose of naloxone and left. Twenty minutes later cardiac arrest occurred. The heart was restarted and she was transferred to the ICU, where she died 5 days later without regaining consciousness.

Possible aspiration of gastric contents

The patient was an obese, heavy smoker. Pregnancy had been complicated by a macrocytic anaemia, for which she was given iron. At Caesarean section for a previous pregnancy she had been noted to be difficult to intubate. She underwent Caesarean section under general anaesthesia after a failed induction of labour. Haemoglobin was 7.8 g/dl. She received 50 mg ranitidine and 100 mg pethidine 2 hours before surgery, and 30 ml of sodium citrate before induction. Laryngoscopy revealed only the arytenoids, but intubation was achieved using a curved stilette. Anaesthesia was uneventful. At the end of the operation, ventilation was inadequate and two doses of atropine and neostigmine were given. The patient was extubated 15 minutes later. Profuse secretions were removed from the pharynx. The patient was transferred to the postnatal ward and some hours later was noticed to be drowsy, 'chesty', tachypnoeic and cyanosed. Arterial oxygen tension was 5.8 kPa on 40% oxygen. She was transferred to a medical ward where she remained for 12 hours before being moved to the ICU. She died 10 days later from ARDS.

Aspiration of gastric contents (late death)

The patient had a prolonged second stage, and had refused epidural analgesia. It was decided that a trial of forceps should be conducted under general anaesthesia. Metoclopramide 10 mg and ranitidine 50 mg were given i.m. and 10 ml of an unspecified antacid given orally. Anaesthesia was induced while a trained assistant applied cricoid pressure. The patient regurgitated a large quantity of gastric contents, and laryngoscopy revealed that some had entered the trachea. Intubation was accomplished easily. After surgery the patient was transferred to the ICU where she died 45 days later, from pneumonia and renal failure.

INDIRECT ANAESTHETIC DEATHS

Obstetric procedure	Cause of death
Emergency unplanned Caesarean section	Haemorrhage; placenta accreta
Laparotomy for ectopic pregnancy	ARDS (haemorrhage)
Surgical termination of pregnancy	Asthma
Emergency unplanned Caesarean section for fetal distress	Bronchopneumonia, renal failure ?aspiration
Emergency unplanned Caesarean section for placental abruption	ARDS (?aspiration)

Emergency planned Caesarean section for fetal distress	Haemorrhage, epidural anaesthesia
Emergency unplanned Caesarean section for eclampsia	ARDS (?aspiration)
Laparotomy for ectopic pregnancy	ARDS (?aspiration)
Laparotomy for tubal pregnancy	Hypoxia ?pulmonary oedema
Elective Caesarean section for pre-eclampsia	Hypoxia ?airway obstruction

RECOMMENDATIONS

- A carbon dioxide analyser should be provided in all locations where general anaesthesia is administered.
- H_2 blockers should be given to all patients who may require anaesthesia, and to those with pre-eclampsia.
- Preoperative emptying of the stomach should be considered where delayed gastric emptying is suspected.
- The stomach should be routinely emptied before extubation.
- When severe blood loss is observed or suspected, a large bore intravenous cannula and a central venous pressure (CVP) line should be inserted, and senior anaesthetic and obstetric assistance sought.
- Guidelines for the provision of blood products should be available in every unit.
- Midwives looking after postoperative patients should be specifically trained in monitoring, airway management and resuscitation. They should be supervised by a defined anaesthetist at all times.
- Monitoring by pulse oximeter should be routine in the early postoperative period.
- Postoperative pain services should be extended to postoperative maternity patients.
- In the interests of facilitating consultant supervision, every effort should be made to bring separate maternity units onto the main hospital site.

Report on Confidential Enquiries into Maternal Deaths in the United Kingdom 1991–93

DEATHS ASSOCIATED WITH ANAESTHESIA

- There were 14 deaths associated with anaesthesia in this triennium: eight deaths were directly attributed to anaesthesia and substandard care was identified in seven of these.
- Hypoxia and airway obstruction were blamed in five cases, ARDS in two and failure of tissue perfusion in one.
- Lack of consultant involvement, inadequate assessment of severity of illness, aspiration of gastric contents, hypovolaemic shock and availability of intensive care facilities were the main factors associated with mortality.
- All direct anaesthetic deaths associated with Caesarean section occurred in women who had general anaesthesia.

DIRECT ANAESTHETIC DEATHS

Haemorrhage, hypoxia, ARDS
A patient underwent laparotomy for ruptured tubal pregnancy. The anaesthetist was an SHO who did not inform the consultant on call. The anaesthetic record was incomplete. Postoperatively the patient became hypoxic, oliguric and moribund, but was not admitted to an ICU until 30 hours after the procedure. She died of cardiopulmonary failure 11 days postoperatively.

- Failure of ward monitoring with pulse oximetry, fluid balance chart or CVP.
- Failure of the anaesthetist to detect the severity of the situation or seek senior assistance.

Post-extubation airway obstruction and cerebral hypoxia
A patient underwent Caesarean section under general anaesthesia, having refused to have the procedure with the existing successful epidural block. She was obese and had poor mouth opening. Anaesthesia was uneventful. After extubation, she developed airway obstruction and, despite repeated attempts, re-intubation was not possible.

- A consultant anaesthetist should have been present for such a high risk case in an isolated unit.
- Extubation was probably premature. Neuromuscular monitoring may have been helpful.
- There was a lack of resident expertise in performing a tracheostomy.

Hypoxia at induction of anaesthesia for Caesarean section
A woman required an elective Caesarean section for unstable lie. She insisted on general anaesthesia. She was induced in the anaesthetic room without monitoring, by a consultant anaesthetist. The patient developed anaphylaxis, which was identified by the anaesthetist after excluding the possibility of misplaced tracheal tube and equipment malfunction. Resuscitation was unsuccessful.

Published in 1996 by HMSO.

Anaesthesia should not have been induced in the anaesthetic room without monitoring.

Tracheal and laryngeal compression causing asphyxia/hypoxia and cardiac arrest

This patient underwent emergency Caesarean section under general anaesthesia for worsening pre-eclampsia. The operation passed uneventfully, but she was returned to theatre to explore the wound which was bleeding. There was other evidence of coagulopathy. Postoperatively, the patient became oliguric and a decision was made to insert an internal jugular line, an attempt at which was unsuccessful, and abandoned. Four hours later the patient developed airway obstruction as a result of neck swelling, and could not be resuscitated.

- The patient should have been monitored with a pulse oximeter.
- Consultants should have been involved.
- ICU admission may have been appropriate after the second operation.
- The decision to use the internal jugular route in a patient with coagulopathy is questionable.

Epidural analgesia (and pulmonary embolism)

A patient was given an epidural for perineal pain 36 hours after forceps delivery. The patient refused to have an intravenous infusion. She was dehydrated and oliguric. After the epidural block, she became pale and vasoconstricted and, later, agitated. She was treated with sedation and frusemide. No oxygen was given. Hypotension progressed to cardiac arrest from which she could not be resuscitated.

Epidural analgesia should have been set up with an intravenous infusion or not at all.

Aspiration of stomach contents

A patient underwent emergency Caesarean section under general anaesthesia for fetal distress. Secretions were noted in the pharynx at intubation. Endobronchial intubation occurred, but was detected and corrected rapidly. There was hypotension and excessive blood loss, but no cross-matched blood was available. O-negative blood was available but not given. She was transferred to the postnatal ward, where her condition deteriorated. She developed ARDS and was transferred to another hospital for intensive care. She died 11 days later. Aspiration of gastric contents was confirmed at autopsy.

- There was inadequate monitoring. A CVP line should have been inserted, and a pulse oximeter used.
- Blood was given too little, too late.
- No consultants were involved until it was too late.

Hypoxia after extubation

An obese patient underwent emergency Caesarean section under general anaesthesia for failure to progress. Intubation was not difficult, but there was severe hypoxia during the operation, despite an adequate capnograph trace. She could not be extubated for 1 hour after the procedure, and then required immediate intubation for stridor. She then arrested, was resuscitated and transferred to HDU for controlled ventilation. She developed multiple organ failure and brain stem death.

A consultant anaesthetist was not informed until too late.

Anaphylaxis to suxamethonium, acute myocardial ischaemia

A patient underwent emergency Caesarean section for fetal distress, under general anaesthesia. Bronchospasm developed after intubation, which was resistant to treatment with adrenaline, and the patient developed bradycardia and died. Post mortem evidence of anaphylaxis to suxamethonium was obtained.

Care was not considered substandard.

DEATHS IN WHICH ANAESTHESIA CONTRIBUTED

Caesarean section for:	Cause of death	Deficiencies
Planned emergency for placenta previa	Acute renal failure, blood loss, coagulopathy	No consultant input. Inadequate blood replacement.
Planned emergency for maternal hypertension	Pulmonary embolus	No consultant input
Planned emergency for pulmonary hypertension	Acute on chronic heart failure, pulmonary hypertension, systemic sclerosis, intrapartum haemorrhage, thrombocytopenic purpura	No physician input
Planned emergency for failure to progress	Postpartum haemorrhage, amniotic fluid embolism	None
Planned emergency for failed induction and intrauterine death	Septicaemia	Antibiotics given late, poor timing of delivery
Planned emergency for fetal distress	Acute right heart failure, primary pulmonary hypertension	Inadequate antenatal investigation.

RECOMMENDATIONS ON ANAESTHESIA AND INTENSIVE CARE

- Facilities for intensive care and high dependency should be conveniently sited and readily available.
- There should be early involvement of consultants in the management of complex deliveries.
- Appropriate monitoring should be available, and training in its use provided.

Report of the Working Group on Specialist Medical Training ('The Calman Report')

> The recommendations of the Chief Medical Officer for changes to the current arrangements for specialist training, in order to comply with EC law.

The recommendations of the Working Group are given in bold type.

EXECUTIVE SUMMARY

This report reviews the current arrangements for specialist training and calls for changes consistent with EC law. It also identifies areas for further review and development.

The report reviews progress with the development of structured and planned training programmes, and notes the potential for the duration of specialist training to be reduced. Based on evidence provided by the Medical Royal Colleges and other educational bodies, it set out the principles to be taken into account in the planning of training programmes. As a result the report recommends:

- *the introduction of improved training programmes by the end of 1995*
- *the establishment of a single training grade by mid 1995 to replace the career registrar and senior registrar grades*
- *the establishment of regular discussions between the educational bodies and the Postgraduate Deans as soon as possible*
- *the introduction of a new Certificate of Completion of Specialist Training (CCST). This will be awarded by the GMC on the advice from the appropriate College that a doctor has completed a training programme which meets the requirements of the EC directives to a standard compatible with independent practice and eligibility for consideration for appointment to a consultant post.*

The report goes on to identify the need for the award of a CCST, or the equivalent qualification from another EC member state, to be shown on the medical register by the introduction of 'CT' as a specialist indicator, together with the relevant specialty, the year of award and the member state in which qualification was awarded.

The implications of these recommendations for the consultant appointment system are noted, and it is recommended that guidance for AAC members should be reconsidered. A number of issues are referred for further consideration to the forum which is to review the operation of the consultant appointments procedure.

The report then considers wider issues arising from the Group's work; first how the UK input into EC medical legislation, and liaison with European colleagues, might be better organised. In particular, it calls for the establishment of improved communication and liaison arrangements, including changes in the membership of the UK dele-

Published in April 1993 by the Department of Health and reproduced with their permission.

gation to the advisory committee on Medical Training. Implications for career structure, manpower planning and service provision are also discussed, in particular the need for increases in the number of consultants.

Finally, the report notes the need for transitional arrangements during the period of change from one system to another and sets out the main strands of action required. It recommends that:

- its recommendation should be implemented within 2 years of being accepted by ministers
- the Chief Medical Officer should monitor the action being taken forward.

BACKGROUND

- The European Commission had expressed concern that the UK's recognition of specialist medical qualifications from other EC member states infringed the 1975 Medical Directive, and had initiated infraction proceedings.
- The Working Group was established by the Health Secretary to consider current arrangements for postgraduate training and scope for harmonisation of specialist training in Europe.
- The Group did not recommend changes to training in general practice.

TRAINING: STRUCTURE, LENGTH AND CONTENT

- Changes in specialist training are founded on three principles:
  1. Specialist training is part of the wider continuum of medical education.
  2. Any changes should ensure standards of training and clinical practice are maintained or improved.
  3. Assessment of trainees should be based on competence.
- The Royal Colleges are already reviewing training programmes, and potential for further improvement has been identified. It should be possible to reduce the minimum length training to 7 years. Lack of career opportunities can prolong time in training posts.
- The Royal Colleges are responsible for deciding the content of training programmes. The Working Group considers that shortening of training can be achieved without compromising standards.
- **Royal Colleges and Faculties should outline training programmes by July 1994, implement them by the end of 1995, and monitor the impact of the changes.**
- General professional or basic specialist training is an important component of the overall continuum of undergraduate and postgraduate education, and a phase of general training should be included in all structured training programmes.
- **The Working Group recommends that the phase of general training should be given further consideration, and be examined by a Working Party convened by the GMC.**
- The end of specialist training will be the award of the CCST. The process for the award of the CCST must be competency based, structured and interactive.
- **The CCST should be awarded by the GMC on advice of the relevant Royal College that the doctor has satisfactorily completed specialist training.**

- Specialist training is part of the continuum of medical education which extends from entry into medical school to the retirement from practice. Arrangements need to take account of the requirements of different specialties, enable doctors in training to exercise choice between specialties and career options, and accommodate the needs of overseas doctors. Entry to training programmes needs to be competitive, and only experience and training which fulfils the requirements of the relevant Royal College will be recognised.
- **'Specialist training' is the period between full registration and award of the CCST. Training programmes need to be flexible enough to allow the trainee's final choice of specialty to be delayed if required.**
- Training has been lengthened in the past because of difficulties in progressing between phases of training. The Group recommends the introduction of a combined career registrar and senior registrar grade as soon as possible. The possibility of replacing the three current grades with a single training grade was considered as a future option.
- **The Health Departments should aim to introduce the combined higher training grade by the end of 1995.**
- The overall responsibility for maintaining standards rests with the Royal Colleges, but both NHS management and Postgraduate Deans have a legitimate interest in the development of structured training.
- **There should be improved dialogue between Medical Royal Colleges, Postgraduate Deans, other educational bodies and NHS management.**

REGISTRATION OF COMPLETION OF SPECIALIST TRAINING

- In the current system, the award of the 'T' indicator by the GMC denotes completion of UK training. This makes no reference to those with qualifications from other EC member states.
- The GMC has agreed to issue a CCST on confirmation by the relevant training body that a doctor has satisfactorily completed a programme which equips him/her for independent practice.
- The adoption of a different indicator such as 'CT' in the medical register to denote award of the CCST, was favoured by the Group. This system would be open to any EC national with appropriate qualifications.
- The length of specialist training in the UK required by the Directives is a minimum specification.
- The Group considered creating a 'restrictive' specialist register to prevent independent practice by those not entered on it. This was not considered necessary at this time in view of the current safeguards.
- **The GMC should award the CCST to trained specialists on the advice of the Royal Colleges, and add 'CT' to their Medical Register Entries. Legislation to implement these changes should be implemented without delay.**

APPOINTMENT TO CONSULTANT

- The current legislation on AACs does not demand any qualifications other than primary medical registration, and does not conflict with EC law.

- Discussions on the consultant appointment system should include guidance for AAC members with regard to EC law. The Group recommends that the consultant appointment process be reviewed.

SPECIALIST TRAINING IN EUROPE

The Health Departments should establish a forum to facilitate the work of members of the Advisory Committee on Medical Training (ACMT), and give further consideration to the membership of the UK delegation to the ACMT.

CAREER STRUCTURE

- The shortening of specialist training may have a significant impact on career structure and workforce arrangements, likely to lead to an increase in the proportion of care provided by consultants.
- A faster expansion of the consultant grade will be needed.
- The clear end point to specialist training will highlight the existence of a 'gap' between the award of the CCST and the appointment to a consultant post. Indefinite continuation in the existing training post would call into question the appropriateness of the work and funding for the job. On the other hand, expecting the doctor to vacate the training post immediately would result in insecurity for the individual concerned and a waste of resources. Proleptic appointments made contingent on the award of the CCST are unlikely to have much impact on the 'gap'.
- A doctor should be able to remain in a training post for a short period after award of the CCST in order to obtain a consultant post. When an individual finally leaves, having failed to get a consultant job, he/she will have the option of retraining in another specialty, working outside the NHS until he/she obtains a consultant post, or obtaining a non-consultant career post.
- **Workforce and career structure issues arising from the implementation of these recommendations should be taken forward within the context of the current review of the implementation of 'Achieving a Balance' (see page 141).**

IMPLEMENTATION AND MONITORING

- The recommendations should be implemented as soon as possible.
- Transitional arrangements will be needed.
- **The Group recommends that a group should be convened whenever necessary by the Chief Medical Officer on behalf of the Health Departments to confirm that appropriate action is being taken forward.**

Implementing the Reforms to Specialist Medical Training PL CMO(95)3

Supplementary document to the 'Calman Report' (see page 121) giving a timetable for the recommended changes.

SUMMARY

1. On 1 December 1995 the new Specialist Registrar grade will be introduced in two vanguard specialties: general surgery and diagnostic radiology.
2. The Specialist Registrar grade, which will replace the career registrar and senior registrar grades, will be formally launched on 1 April 1996. All remaining specialities will enter the transitional stage over the next 12 months.
3. There will be no new appointments to registrar or senior registrar in vanguard specialties after 1 December 1995.
4. A detailed working guidance pack will be available from the NHS Executive.
5. All Regional Health Authorities will be abolished on 1 April 1996, whereupon all specialist trainees will require employment contracts with their local employers.
6. Revised terms and conditions of service will be available for 1 April 1996.
7. Specialist Registrar quotas for each specialty will be issued to Postgraduate Deans. This will mean an increase in some specialties, but no specialty will have a reduced number during the initial period.

Published in October 1995 by the Department of Health.

Specialist Training in Anaesthesia: Supervision and Assessment

Details of the College's proposals for structured training in accordance with the 'Calman Report' (see page 121). In June 1996 it was succeeded by 'Specialist Training in Anaesthesia: Guidelines for Educational Approval' (see page 129).

SUMMARY

- A new 6-year structured training plan which allows an automatic promotion through the stages, provided educational targets are achieved, will shorten training. Trainees already in post will continue to train using the present regulations and service grades.
- The new training plan will be structured. Training should take precedence over service provision. Few hospitals can provide the complete training. Hospital departments are expected to link to form schools of anaesthesia able to provide all aspects of training, including training in the basic sciences. Training has been planned in modules linked to specialties. However, it is recognised that it may be impossible to follow the plan exactly as described. Modules may be taken out of the suggested order or combined. Time allocated to each module is an indicator of the educational weighting.
- The plan includes recommendations for academic content, supervision and assessment.
- The optional year (year '0') may be spent in medical training or other approved elective training at an appropriate time before or during training, but normally before starting years 5 and 6. (A clinical lecturer would be expected to undertake research during this year.)
- One year, including year '0', may be repeated, but it would not count towards the 6-year programme. The training vacancy so created may be used to offer training to trainees from overseas.
- Arrangements for flexible training are described.
- Arrangements for medical officers in the Armed Services are included in the training plan.

THE 10 RULES FOR STRUCTURED TRAINING

1. Clear training objectives.
2. Training must be planned: occurring in college-approved programmes in schools of anaesthesia.
3. Training must be supervised: four levels of supervision are defined.
   - Trainer in the operating theatre or ICU directly supervising or demonstrating techniques.

Published in May 1994 by The Royal College of Anaesthetists.

- Trainer present in the operating theatre suite or ICU available to assist or to advise.
- Trainer available within the hospital.
- Trainer available from outside the hospital as for emergency on call service.

4. Entry criteria: doctors may apply for first and second year training in anaesthesia (BST). Trainees who gain additional experience before entry may have some or all of this time recognised retrospectively.
5. Critical evaluation: including test of knowledge, motor and psychomotor skills. Evaluation policies must be approved by the College.
6. Remedial provision: candidates who fail an examination or assessment may repeat a year.
7. Finite duration.
8. Time is available for study.
9. Individual needs be accommodated: flexible training can be arranged for those with family commitments or for health reasons.
10. Supervisors/trainers have appropriate training and ability.

THE TRAINING PLAN

- Training is defined by year rather than named grade. The modular structure will create a 'national curriculum', facilitating transfer between schools when necessary. Some flexibility in the conducting of the modules is permissible.
- Trainees must register with the College before training begins. A College training number will be given. A national training number (NTN) is given for year 3 onwards by the Postgraduate Dean. More trainees will be enrolled at year 1 than can be accommodated in year 3, to allow for those who enter anaesthesia with different careers in mind.

RECOMMENDED ALLOCATION OF MODULES TO YEARS

- Year 1, selection by interview. Modules 1–4.
- Year 2, satisfactory completion of year 1. Modules 5–9.
- Year 3, selective interview and success in the first part of the examination. Modules 10–16. The final exam may be taken after 30 months in the programme.
- Year '0', may be taken before starting, or at any time during the first 4 years. Intended for experience in research, other disciplines or overseas.
- Year 5, satisfactory completion of years 1–4, plus Fellowship of The Royal College of Anaesthetists (FRCA). Emphasis on organisation, training juniors, management, research/audit, supervised experience.
- Year 6, as for year 5 or a special interest may be taken, for example paeds, cardiac, neuro, etc.

'MAJOR PERVASIVE TOPICS'

- These are topics pertinent to all modules and continued throughout training. The list includes identifying the difficult airway, checking equipment, understanding cardiopulmonary resuscitation (CPR), etc.

MODULES

1. Introduction to anaesthesia (24 weeks). Supervision level 1 for first 12 weeks, level 1 and 2 for following 12 weeks.
2. A: anaesthesia for ENT surgery (4 weeks).
   B: anaesthesia for dental surgery (4 weeks).
   Level 1 supervision initially, and for ASA 3+ patients or children under 10.
3. Anaesthesia for gynaecology and urology (12 weeks). Supervision level 2 or 3, 1 for techniques not previously taught.
4. Recovery/HDU/acute pain (4 weeks) supervision level 3 and 4.
5. A: initial ICU training. An ICU will not be recognised unless there is a nominated consultant with protected sessions for ITU.
   B: resuscitation, including competence in ATLS, ALS and APLS.
   Twelve weeks A and B.
6. Obstetric analgesia and anaesthesia (12 weeks). The unit should have one consultant session per 500 deliveries per annum, full time cover above 3000 deliveries. Supervision level 1 for first 8 weeks, level 2 for 4 weeks. Experience should include at least 50 lumbar epidurals and 20 general anaesthetics for obstetric management.
7. Anaesthesia for trauma and orthopaedics (12 weeks).
8. Anaesthesia for general surgery and major vascular surgery (12 weeks). Initial supervision level 1 and 2, progressing to 3 when tutor has confidence in the trainee's ability.
9. Ophthalmic anaesthesia (4 weeks). Supervision level 1 progressing to 2 or 3.
10. Paediatric anaesthesia (12 weeks). Level 1 supervision for all children under 3 and for at least 50% of children over 3.
11. Day-stay anaesthesia (8 weeks). Supervision level 1, subsequently level 2.
12. A: anaesthesia for plastic surgery.
    B: care of the burned patient.
    Four weeks. Supervision 1 and 2.
13. Anaesthesia for neurosurgery (4 weeks). Supervision level 1.
14. Anaesthesia for cardiothoracic surgery (4 weeks). Supervision level 1.
15. Anaesthesia and sedation for neuroradiology (4 weeks). Supervision levels 1 and 2.
16. Care for those with chronic pain (4 weeks). Supervision level 1.
17. Academic module (4 weeks). To promote understanding of the scientific basis of anaesthetic practice, learn scientific skills such as planning a study, statistics, presentation skills, etc. There should be a weekly academic day during further training.
18. Year 5 (12 months). General clinical and management training.
19. Year 6 (12 months). General clinical training or training in specialised anaesthesia.

Military medicine training module
The services may require the trainee to undertake general duties for 2 years, which may be recognised as year '0' depending on supervision. A break in training between years 3 and 5 would be permitted.

Specialist Training in Anaesthesia: Guidelines for Educational Approval

Lays down standards for Royal College approval of training posts in anaesthesia.

GENERAL

Training posts will only receive Royal College approval if they comply with educational requirements and are part of an approved training programme.

THE SCHOOL OF ANAESTHESIA

- All hospitals within a School of Anaesthesia must agree to regular reviews of training.
- The number of approved posts will be agreed by the Royal College of Anaesthetists (RCA) Training Committee.
- Training programmes should require rotation through at least two hospitals.
- Hospitals within a school will in general be expected to offer experience in a range of basic anaesthetic specialties.
- Hospitals seeking to train specialist registrars will in addition be required to provide one or more modules of specialised experience, for example cardiothoracic, neurosurgery, etc.
- Single-specialty hospitals may be attached to Schools of Anaesthesia, in order to complement the overall training.
- Standards imposed by the RCA, the Association of Anaesthetists of Great Britain and Ireland, the King's Fund and NCEPOD should be adhered to.
- Participating hospitals must have adequate staffing to meet its service needs.
- There must be adequate supervision by an appropriate number of consultants.
- Non-consultant career grade staff who possess the FRCA may participate in supervision of trainees.
- There should be trained dedicated skilled assistance for all anaesthetists at all times.
- SHO work should be supervised, at a level determined by local assessment.
- Consultants and others involved in teaching must fulfil the RCA CME requirements.
- Trainees in intensive care should have the opportunity for continuity of care by a modular attachment.
- Education and training must be provided, and records of attendance at teaching sessions must be kept.
- Log books are mandatory for trainees.
- Assessment of trainee progress must be reviewed regularly. Trainees must have a mechanism to assess their programme.
- There should be appropriate departmental facilities.

Published in June 1996 by The Royal College of Anaesthetists.

- All patients should be seen preoperatively and postoperatively by an anaesthetist, preferably the one responsible for the anaesthetic.
- There should be an emergency theatre available 24 hours a day, but out-of-hours operating must be kept to an absolute minimum.
- Monitoring and checking of equipment should comply with the recommendations of the Association of Anaesthetists of Great Britain and Ireland (see page 44).
- Anaesthetic records should comply with RCA guidelines (see page 48).
- A properly staffed and equipped recovery room must be available 24 hours a day, supported by access to high dependency and/or intensive care facilities.
- Trainees should not cover ICU, obstetrics or pain management services without consultant supervision being readily available.
- The department should have a full range of educational facilities available.
- Departmental policies on pain management, resuscitation, etc. should be clearly written and updated.
- On call accommodation should comply with Postgraduate Deans' recommendations.

Specialist Training for Senior House Officers in Anaesthesia

Sets out the way in which the training principles detailed in 'Specialist Training in Anaesthesia, Supervision and Assessment' (see page 126) can be applied to the first 2 years of training.

INTRODUCTION

- SHO posts should be linked in a training rotation where possible.
- Where existing SHO training schemes conform to these basic principles, the College does not seek to impose an alternative system.
- Self-directed learning, with access to a full range of information resources, supplemented with appropriate supervision, is of paramount importance.
- The principles of training are that it should
  - have clear objectives
  - be planned
  - be supervised
  - be evaluated
  - allow time for personal study
  - accommodate specific needs of individuals
  - be of finite duration.
- The aims of SHO training are:
  - to provide wide clinical experience
  - to encourage personal and professional development
  - to enable the trainee to progress to the next stage at the appropriate time
  - to develop an interest and knowledge of audit and research.

Logbooks

- The trainee **must** maintain a logbook throughout his/her training, either written or electronic.
- The logbook will be analysed to assess individual training, or to assess the training programme.
- It is acknowledged that two aspects of training are not easily monitored with a logbook: the ability to modify anaesthetic technique according to individual medical condition, and the ability to communicate effectively with patients, relatives and other staff.

THE INTRODUCTORY SIX MONTHS

- Objectives are 'the basic principles of safe and effective anaesthesia, resuscitation, and both the prevention and treatment of pain', with emphasis on the role of the anaesthetist in perioperative care.

Published in 1996 by The Royal College of Anaesthetists.

- Every trainee should register with the College within a few days of commencing their post.
- Supervision should be level 1 during the first 12 weeks, with level 2 in the following 12 weeks at the trainer's discretion.

A comprehensive list of specific educational and practical skills to be taught is included.

TRAINING FOR THE NEXT 18 MONTHS

During this period, trainees should acquire sufficient knowledge and experience to pass the primary FRCA, and become eligible for appointment as a specialist registrar. By the end of this stage, SHOs should be able to:

- undertake anaesthesia for most routine cases
- assist in anaesthetic care of complex cases
- provide anaesthetic care for routine obstetrics
- organise, with the surgical team, the emergency list; identify potential problems and seek appropriate help
- understand the principles underlying the care of patients in intensive care and high dependency units
- understand the principles of pain management
- participate in audit
- pass the primary FRCA.

SHOs should have experience in all areas except neonatal, cardiothoracic and neurological surgery.

(A comprehensive list for guidance to the required practical experience is included.)

ASSESSMENT OF SHOS IN ANAESTHESIA

Continuous assessment of trainees was an integral part of the Calman proposals (see page 121).

There is some confusion about terminology:

Formative assessment is a retrospective, usually informal process, belonging to the trainee, and for the trainee's benefit.

Summative assessment is a formal and more complex process, to assess whether the trainee has reached specified standards, quantify experience and estimate eligibility to progress. Summative assessment is primarily for the benefit of the assessor.

Appraisal is 'a review of an individual's strengths and weaknesses, enabling the construction of a plan to develop new skills and enhance existing ones'. This should be restricted to the prospective process of planning a trainee's educational and clinical training.

Formative assessment
- Should be the responsibility of a designated educational supervisor, usually a College tutor.

- Should be conducted at the end of the first 6 months, and the end of the first year.
- Should be informal and directed at finding out the trainee's personal view of the training programme.
- Should reach agreed, written, detailed conclusions, which are confidential to trainee and supervisor.

Summative assessment
- This is intended to formally recognise that SHOs have achieved the criteria for entry into the SpR grade.
- Should be carried out at the end of the second year.

Those who do not meet the requirements may:

- continue into a third year (SHO3) funded by the Postgraduate Dean
- enter a different specialty or a general practice scheme.

Those who do meet the criteria have the options to:

- be appointed to an SpR post, by competitive interview, and obtain a NTN
- remain in SHO3, pending suitable vacancies at SpR grade
- enter an externally funded post, for example research fellowship or training abroad.

Further summative assessments should be unnecessary, except where a long absence from training has been taken (e.g. to raise a family). In this case, assessments are carried out by the Postgraduate Dean or Regional Adviser.

Continuing Medical Education: Report of a Working Party

College recommendations for a system of accreditation for activities of continuing medical education (CME).

EXECUTIVE SUMMARY

1. *RCA recommends CME as an essential part of professional practice for all career anaesthetists.*
2. *Participation on CME will be assessed by a system of cognate points. Reaccreditation at 5 year intervals is recommended.*
3. *RCA will keep a register of fellows in good standing who maintain their accreditation status; such fellows will be eligible to be 'designated teachers'. This register will be available for public inspection.*
4. *Failure to obtain an adequate number of cognate points in each 5 year cycle will result in loss of designated teacher eligibility.*
5. *Hospital accreditation will be dependent upon at least 80% of the consultant members of an anaesthetic department possessing designated teacher status. Only designated teachers will be regarded as suitable to educate trainee anaesthetists.*
6. *RCA would welcome and encourage proposals from the GMC to institute mandatory five yearly re-registration of specialist status on the Medical Register. The RCA proposals for reaccreditation contained in the document could provide the basis for such re-registration.*
7. *The CME proposals will require the establishment of a Department of Education within the RCA with a director who will require support and assistance for tracking the CME status of all specialist anaesthetists within the UK.*

INTRODUCTION

Possession of a specialist qualification does not equip individuals with all the skills and knowledge required throughout a professional life. Not all anaesthetists make conscientious efforts to keep up to date, and the solitary working environment of most senior anaesthetists compounds the problem. This document contains the recommendations of the RCA on CME and applies to all career grades in anaesthesia.

BACKGROUND TO CME

CME has been discussed within the College since 1990. Several principles have emerged. The RCA supports a system of CME, and wishes it to extend to all anaesthetists regardless of grade or status. A 5-year cycle of accreditation is favoured,

Published in July 1993 by The Royal College of Anaesthetists and the Executive Summary is reproduced with their permission.

mandatory re-examination is not. Careful consideration must be given to cost implications.

TYPES OF CME AVAILABLE

1. **Personal reading** of books and journals is an important part of CME, but cannot be accepted without an effective means of audit. Wide reading is encouraged, but there is a category of essential reading, for example the latest guidelines on cardiopulmonary resuscitation.
2. **Local meetings**, for example journal clubs, audit meetings, grand rounds, etc., should be assessed as part of a hospital accreditation visit by the College.
3. **Regional societies**.
4. **National and international courses and lectures**.
5. **Clinical scenarios**.
6. **Visits to other centres.** Consultants should have the opportunity to work together occasionally, in order to pass on techniques.
7. **Visiting lecturers**.
8. **Teaching** activity should carry bonus points in a system for evaluating CME.
9. **Research and writing**, provided it is published, should score highly for CME.
10. **Higher degrees**.
11. **Supervision of higher degrees**.
12. **Practical or 'hands-on' skill**, for example satisfactory completion of an ATLS course.

CME PROPOSALS OF THE ROYAL COLLEGE OF ANAESTHETISTS

The RCA regards CME as essential, and considers that the cognate points system is a satisfactory way to start recognition.

The RCA proposes that those who have completed CME satisfactorily within a 5-year span should receive a certificate and be included on a publicly available list.

The RCA proposes to develop a points system for all CME activities, and arrange it so that the majority of anaesthetists 'pass' with their present activities. In the long term, the quality of CME activities and the effect of implementation of CME should be audited.

Cognate point scoring scheme

Self-learning

Personal reading	1 point/hour
Clinical scenarios	1 point/hour
Visits to other centres	1 point/hour
Preparation of lectures	10 points
Editing a book	25 points
Original research	20 points
Review articles	20 points
Chapters	10 points
Case reports	5 points
Editorials	10 points
MD, MSc or PhD thesis	50 points
Monograph (>15 000 words)	50 points
Completion of ATLS, etc.	10 points
Maximum in 5 years	150

Audience participation in CME meetings

Maximum in 5 years	150

Locally organised meetings 1 point per hour

Maximum in 5 years	150

Total needed in 5 years 250

IMPLEMENTATION OF CME. THE NEED FOR A SANCTION

The minority of anaesthetists that currently fail to participate in CME is unlikely to accept a formal programme recommended by the RCA unless there are sanctions.

When anaesthetists fail to maintain accreditations they **cannot be recognised as a teacher** by the RCA, and should not be allocated anaesthetists for training. As part of training programme recognition, the RCA should consider the proportion of accredited designated teachers within a department.

FINANCIAL IMPLICATIONS

There will be substantial additional costs for the following reasons:

1. All consultants will be encouraged to make full use of their allocation of funded study leave
2. Implementation of CME will require a central education officer based in the RCA
3. There are financial implications to such activities as, for example, anaesthetists spending time in other departments.

Implementation of Proposals for Continuing Medical Education

> This document suggests a framework for the implemetation of CME proposals outlined in 'Continuing Medical Education: Report of a Working Party'
> (see page 134).

INTRODUCTION

Following the publication by the RCA of a Working Party report on CME, the College undertook a pilot study to test the proposals. The survey showed that the majority of anaesthetists would easily meet the target of 250 credits in 5 years.

In 1994 the Directors of CME from all the Royal Colleges agreed the following.

1. There should be as much commonality as possible between the Colleges' activities.
2. There would be a 2 year introductory phase.
3. The basic unit of activity should be 1 hour, equating to one credit. A study day will be five credits and a half-day three credits.
4. There should be an appropriate mix between internal and external activities.
5. The cycle of CME activity and assessment should last 5 years.

The RCA does not regard the function of CME as ascertaining an individual's fitness to practice.

SCHEME FOR IMPLEMENTATION OF CME

The proposed scheme is intended to be as simple and inexpensive as possible, while allowing verification, and achieving as much commonality as possible with other Colleges. The scheme will apply to all anaesthetists in non-training posts.

CATEGORISATION OF ACTIVITIES

There are two categories of CME activities: internal and external.

External activities
1. Attendance at RCA educational meetings: scoring 5 for one study day, 3 for a half-day.
2. Other meetings
- Automatically approved: for example Association meetings, Royal Society of Medicine, some regional meetings. A list of 'approved' providers could be kept by the College.
- Individually approved provision of CME. For a meeting to gain approval, the final programme must be sent to the regional co-ordinator (regional) or RCA (national). Approval will not be given retrospectively.

Published in April 1995 by The Royal College of Anaesthetists.

At present, meetings must all be educational, formal, structured and scheduled. Records of attendance should be kept.

Internal activities

Hospital-based

Case conferences	1 credit/hour
Audit meetings	1 credit/hour
Journal clubs	1 credit/hour
Attendance at formal lectures	1 credit/hour

Self-learning

Visit to another centre	5 credits for a day, 3 for half a day
Preparation of lecture	5 credits per lecture
Editing a book, chapter in a book, paper, review article, case report, editorial, monograph	5 credits per publication
ATLS, ACLS, ALS, APLS, PALS, PHEC, PHTLS	5 credits each.

Other academic activities may be included by the RCA.

IMPLEMENTATION OF CME

It is necessary to verify CME activities, and the College proposes a system of random verification.

Plan
1. **Log books** of CME activity should be kept by all permanent grade anaesthetists.
2. **A local co-ordinator** should be nominated by each unit. His/her task will be to ensure that the College receives a description of the credit points obtained by members of the department.
3. **The regional co-ordinator**/REA will approve regional meetings for CME.
4. **The Royal College of Anaesthetists** will:
   * issue a list of CME-approved meetings
   * maintain a database of the CME status of all non-trainee anaesthetists
   * inspect log books during accreditation visits
   * arrange a random check on the status of individuals.

Timetable
April 1995   All non-training grade staff should maintain a record of their CME activities.

April 1996   Local co-ordinators should submit a list of all permanent staff with an indication of their CME credits

April 2000   The College calculates the CME status of anaesthetists, who should have reached 250 credits by this time.

Departments where more than 20% of consultants have failed to reach the CME requirements are likely to lose recognition for training purposes.

Individual consultants who fail to obtain 250 credits will not be designated as college teachers, and should not be allocated trainee anaesthetists.

Achieving a Balance

Proposals for changes to training grade and consultant numbers, in order to match the numbers of posts with expected vacancies.

MAIN PROPOSALS

- Expansion of consultant posts in line with existing plans produced by Health Authorities.
- One hundred new consultant posts in General Medicine, General Surgery and Orthopaedics, 45 in 1987–88, 55 in 1998–89.
- Conversion of registrar and senior registrar posts that are surplus to requirements to consultant posts where justified on service grounds.
- Schemes for early retirement to facilitate proposed changes in staffing structure.
- Continuation of joint planning for senior registrar posts, with regional quotas relating to expected consultant vacancies.
- Designation of registrars as 'career' or 'visiting'.
- Setting of quotas for the numbers of career registrars, relating them to senior registrar numbers.
- Registrar contracts to be held at region.
- An overall reduction in registrar numbers.
- Relaxation of the ceiling for SHO numbers, and arrangements to monitor their supply and demand.
- Careers advice and counselling for SHOs.
- Two extra incremental points on the SHO scale.
- Introduction of a new non-training career grade (Staff grade), with strict manpower controls.
- Arrangements for regrading from Staff grade to Associate Specialist, or vice versa.
- After introduction of the Staff grade, no further appointments to clinical assistant posts of six sessions or more.
- Consultants in acute specialties will have to accept greater direct involvement in patient care, but their middle-grade supporting staff should not fall below an acceptable level in number. Health Authorities will review the staffing levels required in acute units.
- Mechanisms to identify and help 'stuck doctors'.
- The Steering group will continue to monitor all aspects of 'achieving a balance' carefully.
- In the long term, the length of time spent in registrar and senior registrar grades should be reduced, and the two grades should eventually be merged.
- All stages of implementation should be under way by the end of 1988, but completion of the programme may take many years.

Published in October 1987 by The Steering Group for Implementation on behalf of the UK Health Departments, the Joint Consultants Committee and Chairmen of Regional Health Authorities.

Anaesthetic Agents:
Controlling Exposure under COSHH

Advice about monitoring and control of exposure to inhaled anaesthetic agents, in accordance with Control of Substances Hazardous to Health (COSHH) regulations.

INTRODUCTION

The possible risk to health from repeated exposure to anaesthetic agents has been a concern for some time. The Health and Safety Commission's Advisory Committee on Toxic Substances (ACTS) has concluded that there may be risk from persistently high exposure, but levels could be identified which pose no threat. The ACTS recommended occupational exposure standards (OESs)

The OESs for anaesthetic agents which come into force in 1996 are

Nitrous oxide	100 p.p.m.
Enflurane	50 p.p.m.
Isoflurane	50 p.p.m.
Halothane	10 p.p.m.

Measured over an 8 hour time-weighted average reference period.

EFFECTS OF EXPOSURE TO ANAESTHETIC AGENTS

Particular concern has been raised over the possibility of an increased rate of miscarriage.

Nitrous oxide
There is no convincing human evidence that exposure to nitrous oxide in the workplace has caused any fetal abnormalities or any other health effects. Fetal abnormalities are seen in rats given 1000 p.p.m. for 8 hours a day, but not in those given 500 p.p.m.

Volatile agents
Again, no human evidence exists to suggest adverse reproductive effects. Animal studies have demonstrated adverse effects during exposures to 1000 p.p.m. or more. Levels of 100 p.p.m. for halothane and 600 p.p.m. for isoflurane have not been shown to cause animal effects. Enflurane is the least toxic.

Published in 1995 by The Health Services Advisory Committee.

The levels chosen for the OESs are therefore well below levels which have been shown to be safe in animals.

THE CONTROL OF SUBSTANCES HAZARDOUS TO HEALTH (COSHH) REGULATIONS 1994

This set out the legal requirements for protecting the health of people in the workplace from hazardous substances, including anaesthetic agents. It requires employers to reduce exposure by inhalation to the OESs.

Trade union safety representatives must be consulted by employers, to assist in the development of control measures.

ADVICE ON COMPLYING WITH KEY ASPECTS OF THE COSHH REGULATIONS

Assessing risk to health
'Action checklist'

- Where is exposure likely to occur?
- Who is likely to be exposed?
- Estimate exposure.
- Compare exposure with the OESs.
- If exposures exceed or are likely to exceed OESs, decide what control measures are required.
- Review assessment regularly.

How to estimate exposure
Operating theatre: 'action checklist'

- For what period of time are staff exposed?
- Is there a scavenging system in place?
- How effective is the ventilation?
- Is there any leakage from anaesthetic equipment, breathing circuit or scavenging into the operating theatre?
- Is the gas flow turned off when not in use?
- Are vaporizers filled in ventilated areas or filled and drained with 'keyed filling devices'?

If you are using active scavenging to BS 6834:1994, and (room) ventilation complies with HTM 2025 and HBN 26, and there is no significant leakage from the anaesthetic system, then it is unlikely that you will exceed the OESs.

Inhalation analgesia in obstetrics and dentistry: 'action checklist'

- For what period of time are staff exposed?
- How well is the room ventilated?

When nitrous oxide is used as an analgesic, staff may be exposed to high concentrations, but if this is for short periods, OESs are unlikely to be exceeded.

Recovery rooms: 'action checklist'

- For what period of time are staff exposed?
- How well is the room ventilated?

Measuring exposure

If you cannot easily estimate exposure, you may need to carry out personal sampling. You will not need to measure each agent separately, provided you do not use volatile agents in the absence of nitrous oxide. Adequate control of nitrous oxide generally implies adequate control of other agents.

Regular review is required, and intervals of 5 years are recommended. It is good practice to keep a record of assessments.

Maintenance and testing of control measures

Control measure should be examined and tested at suitable intervals. Function of scavenging and ventilation should be checked at least once a week, and serviced according to the manufacturer's recommendations (at least every 14 months).

Monitoring exposure at the workplace

A programme of routine monitoring of exposure is not normally necessary. Consider monitoring if:

- you think control measures may be inadequate
- you change your working practices
- your COSHH assessment shows wide variations in exposure.

How to sample

Personal exposure levels can be determined by taking time-weighted air samples in the breathing zone of those potentially most exposed. The most cost-effective method uses small diffusive samplers attached to clothing.

Informing and training employees
- Make sure your employees know the possible risks to their health of exposure to anaesthetic gases and volatile agents.
- Make sure your employees understand the need for control measures.
- Make sure your employees understand the correct use of control measures.
- Provide information to the employees on the results of any monitoring.

Recommended control measures
1. **General anaesthesia**: scavenging systems must conform to BS 6834:1994. Further guidance is given in HTM 2022. Passive and semi-passive scavenging may not control exposure to OESs.
2. **Ventilation**, when adequate, reduces exposure by diluting anaesthetic gases in the operating theatre. Advice is available in HBN 26 and HTM 2025.
3. **Obstetrics**: exposure control relies on good housekeeping and ventilation. HBN 21 recommends that balanced supply and extract ventilation is provided at six to seven air changes per hour.

4. **Recovery areas**: the major source of pollution is the patient's exhaled breath. Exposure control relies on ventilation. Fifteen air changes per hour are recommended, with the supply air terminal placed above the recovery bed positions.

Anaesthetic-related Equipment: Purchase, Maintenance and Replacement

Advice on the management of anaesthetic equipment.

SUMMARY

1. *Each directorate should nominate one consultant with responsibility for equipment management and liaising with the manager of technical servicing.*
2. *Anaesthetic equipment used in some locations may have shared use. An inventory should be kept and management responsibilities should be clearly defined for all equipment for which the anaesthetic department is responsible.*
3. *A separate capital asset register which includes equipment paid for by charities is required for depreciation and replacement purposes.*
4. *The nominated consultant must be aware of current legislation in the UK and Ireland. There are also relevant European directives being developed.*
5. *A planned preventative maintenance programme is essential. Quality issues must be monitored.*
6. *There should be a departmental policy for equipment breakdown.*
7. *A planned replacement programme which defines equipment life and disposal procedures should be agreed.*
8. *Purchase of equipment involves wide consultation and technical advice is essential to ensure practicability and cost-effectiveness.*
9. *Use of private capital must be carefully considered.*
10. *An acceptance procedure and training programme should be part of a safety protocol.*

Published in February 1994 by The Association of Anaesthetists of Great Britain and Ireland and reproduced with their permission.

Report of the Working Party on Guidelines for Sedation by Non-anaesthetists

Standards from The Royal College of Surgeons on the safe conduct of sedation in the absence of an anaesthetist.

STANDARDS

- Communication must be maintained with the patient during sedation.
- The risks in each case should be assessed before the procedure by the sedationist.
- There must be a table with head-down tilt, oxygen, suction and resuscitation equipment immediately available.
- When carefully titrated, intravenous benzodiazepines have a suitable safety margin. Midazolam is the drug of choice.
- Nitrous oxide is suitable for inhalational sedation.
- Opioids enhance the effect of benzodiazepines. Failure to modify the doses of these drugs when used in combination may be hazardous.
- Specific antagonists naloxone and flumazenil should be immediately available, but should not encourage a lax attitude to titrating dose against response.
- Every sedated patient should receive oxygen-enriched air.
- Where the sedationist is also the operator, at least one other trained person should be present to monitor the patient.
- All patients receiving sedation should have an intravenous cannula, left in place until after recovery.
- The management of children undergoing sedation in hospital is a specialised field requiring its own standards of patient care.
- Staff of all grades should be familiar with resuscitation.
- Clinical monitoring must be continuous until recovery is complete.
- Minimum criteria for discharge including stable vital signs, ability to walk without support, toleration of oral fluids, the ability to void urine, minimal nausea, adequate analgesia and appropriate aftercare.
- Day cases should be accompanied home by a responsible adult, who should be given written instructions. The patient should not be allowed to sign legally binding agreements, drive or carry out any activity involving motor skills for 24 hours after intravenous sedation.

Published in June 1993 by The Royal College of Surgeons of England.

Assessing the Effects of Health Technologies: Principles, Practice, Proposals

Advice from the Department of Health on the adoption of new technologies into clinical practice.

MAIN POINTS AND RECOMMENDATIONS

Outcomes for evaluating the effects of health technologies

a) *It will often be desirable to assess the effects of a technology in terms of a range of possible outcome measures, including mortality, clinical measures of morbidity, and psychological, social and economic outcomes. Although it may be necessary to decide whether to adopt a new technology on the basis of evidence about its short-term effects, assessing its effects in the longer term may also be important.*

b) *Because some outcomes are rare and others frequent, obtaining a broad and reasonably complete picture of the effects of a technology may require a number of interrelated studies using appropriate methods and sample sizes. It is often inappropriate to try to examine a wide variety of outcomes within the same study.*

c) *The impact of a technology on other services, and on society, should be studied to provide information for policy and managerial decisions, and for public debate.*

Research designs for evaluating the effects of health technologies

a) *Reliable assessment of the effects of a technology requires both that systematic errors (biases) and that random errors (the play of chances) should be small in comparison with the size of effect that is realistic to expect from the technology being evaluated.*

b) *Analyses of observational data can be used to demonstrate the effects of health technologies when these effects are large, and in some circumstances in which randomised trials are not feasible. They should also be used to expose important uncertainty about the effectiveness of technologies, and to facilitate the design of randomised trials.*

c) *Randomised trials of sufficient size should be performed to detect important beneficial or harmful effects of existing health technologies when their effects are in doubt, and to assess recently introduced technologies, the effects of which are unknown.*

d) *A mixture of qualitative and quantitative research is often required to study unanticipated 'knock-on' effects of introducing an effective health technology, both on the health services, and more widely.*

Using evidence about the effects of health technologies

a) *Existing evidence about the effects of health technologies should be reviewed systematically, using methods which reduce biases and random errors. Without more systematically conducted reviews of existing evidence about the effects of technologies – including systematic*

Published by the Department of Health Research and Development Division and reproduced with their permission.

overviews (meta-analyses) when appropriate – policies for health care and health services research will remain inadequately informed.

b) The results of methodologically sound reviews of the effects of health technologies should be synthesised appropriately and then disseminated in forms that a wide variety of decision makers, including patients, can understand.

c) For various reasons, research evidence about the effects of health technologies is not used. Sometimes the evidence is not sufficiently strong to be convincing; sometimes the results are inconvenient or incompatible with strongly held beliefs. In circumstances in which strong evidence is available, careful consideration needs to be given to the development of mechanisms to ensure the research findings are reflected in appropriate health care practices.

Fostering proper assessment of the effects of health technologies for the NHS

a) Information about completed and current research assessing the effects of health technologies, in Britain and abroad, should be assembled in easily consulted, up-to-date databases that are easily accessible to clinicians and managers. Funds are needed to allow researchers to devote the time required to conduct reviews which respect scientific principles, and to update these reviews efficiently as new evidence becomes available.

b) Proposals for new research to evaluate the effects of health technologies should always take into account the results of systematic reviews of existing evidence.

c) A central dissemination unit is needed to prepare materials (not necessarily only in writing) about the effects of health technologies, and to ensure their wide dissemination to relevant target audiences.

d) Unevaluated forms of care which have been adopted in the NHS should be paid for whether or not they are being offered within a research project. A strong case, however, can be made for ensuring that unevaluated forms of care are paid for by the NHS only if they are offered as part of properly designed research to assess their effects.

e) Research centres are needed to help assemble registers of relevant published, unpublished and ongoing studies, to simulate, coordinate and assist those reviewing evidence on the effects of health technologies, and to contribute to new research. These centres might focus either on a priority area of health care, or on particular research methods.

f) Efficient health technology assessment for the NHS, by capable and knowledgeable people, requires a career structure for those who wish to specialise in this work. Urgent consideration needs to be given to training and career provision for those needed to undertake the work that the NHS Research and Development Programme is seeking to promote.

g) Various obstacles, relating to informed consent, corporate identity and costs of treatment, often prevent clinicians from taking part in research to assess technologies. These obstacles must be acknowledged more explicitly and overcome.

Supporting Research and Development in the NHS: A Report to the Minister for Health by a Research and Development Task Force Chaired by Professor Anthony Culyer ('The Culyer Report')

> A report on changes to the organisation of funding for research and development in the NHS.

KEY RECOMMENDATIONS:

- A national forum should be created, chaired by the Director of Research and Development (R&D), to exchange information about the research strategies of the national bodies which sponsor or support R&D in the NHS.
- The Central Research and Development Committee (CRDC) should be recast to provide advice to the Director of R&D on all issues relating to R&D which have implications for NHS funding.
- The membership of the CRDC should be reviewed to ensure that the perspectives of NHS purchasers and providers and of key commissioners of R&D are adequately represented
- The terms on which the NHS provides service support to the Medical Research Council should be reviewed.
- The Regional Offices' Directors of R&D (RDRDs)should be the focal point for R&D within each region. Each RDRD should lead a consultative body to identify research priorities for the region. RDRDs should also have a role in commissioning and managing R&D.
- The NHS should develop and publish principles and criteria guiding the use of NHS funds related to R&D.
- With effect from 1995/1996, a single explicit funding stream should replace the current diverse funding mechanisms, including the Research part of the Service Increment for Teaching and Research (SIFTR), the non-SIFTR scheme and others.
- This funding stream should be conceived as a levy on all health care purchasers' allocations, and determined annually.
- The direct, indirect and service cost of R&D in NHS providers, currently funded from patients care income, should be declared and added to the amount levied on purchasers' allocations.
- Purchasers of health care should allow providers freedom to support pre-protocol work, curiosity-driven research, etc., and fund them where costs are not met by external sponsors.
- Purchasers and providers should be able to supplement the levy in order to meet national and regional priorities more quickly.

Published in September 1994 by HMSO.

- The R&D-related funding of the NHS should be viewed in three categories:
  1. Direct and indirect costs of R&D projects
  2. Service costs of individual projects whether the project is commissioned by the NHS or sponsored externally
  3. Cost of maintaining particular research facilities and staff that are not attributable to any specific project.
- To decide which centres should receive funding for research facilities costs, there should be a formalised assessment by research ratings, like those used by the Higher Educational Funding Council for England. There should be a full review every 3–5 years.
- The NHS executive should develop and publish a statement of the broad scope of research facilities funding and the internal systems for business planning, monitoring and accountability required to secure it.
- The NHS executive should develop criteria for research facilities funding, and interim costing techniques for research, for use during 1995–96.
- Changes to current funding should be phased in over an agreed period.
- Funds for service support and direct costs of R&D should be available to primary and community health professionals.
- There should be R&D commissioning units, accountable to the Director of R&D through the NHS Executive's Regional Offices.
- All significant R&D should be captured on a national database.
- The NHS Executive should develop and publish methodologies, following common principles, for costing and accounting for R&D-related activities in secondary, primary and community care settings.
- A human resource strategy for R&D in the NHS should be developed, embracing training and more general personnel issues.

Accident and Emergency

Medical staffing of accident and emergency services. *British Medical Association Joint Consultants Committee 1978.*

Audit

Audit & quality in anaesthesia. Summary of a one day meeting held 9 December 1993. *The Royal College of Anaesthetists.*

Audit and the purchaser/provider interaction. *Report of a Working Group of the Regional Medical Audit Coordinators' Committee and Conference of Colleges' Audit Working Group Members 1993.*

Audit in anaesthesia and Quality of Practice Committee. *The Royal College of Anaesthetists 1993.*

Audit in anaesthesia and Quality of Practice. *The Royal College of Anaesthetists 1993.*

Audit in anaesthesia: results of a survey by questionnaire. *Quality of Practice Committee, Royal College of Anaesthetists 1991/2.*

Clinical audit and Quality of Practice in anaesthesia. *The Royal College of Anaesthetists.*

Meeting and improving standards in health care – a policy statement on the development of clinical audit, EL(93)59. *NHS Executive.*

Organisational audit (accreditation UK) anaesthetic services. *King's Fund 1992.*

Children and Neonates

Surgical services for the newborn. *The Royal College of Surgeons of England.*

Report on the occurrence of pain and disability in adults and children in the UK. *K. Budd, Quality of Practice Committee, Royal College of Anaesthetists.*

Working Party on organ transplantation in neonates. *Conference of Medical Royal Colleges in UK.*

Children first. A study of hospital services. *Audit Commission 1993 HMSO.*

Quality review: setting standards for children in health care. *C. Hogg, National Association for Welfare of Children in Hospital.*

Consultants terms and conditions

Consultants distinction awards. *Department of Health Welsh Office.*

Consultants' guide for the 90's. *BMA Central Consultants and Specialists Committee.*

Critical incidents, risk management

Critical incident reporting in anaesthesia: a report of a pilot scheme at the Hammersmith Hospital. *Imrie, Powell and Lumley. Quality of Practice Committee, Royal College of Anaesthetists.*

Safeguards against failure to remove swabs and instruments from patients. *The Medical Defence Union and The Royal College of Nursing.*

Safeguards against wrong operations. *The Medical Defence Union and The Royal College of Nursing.*

Risk management in day unit surgery. *The Medical Defence Union.*

Day surgery

Measuring quality: the patient's view of day surgery. *Audit Commission 1992.*
All in a day's work: an audit of day surgery in England & Wales. *Audit Commission 1992.*

Guidelines for day case surgery. *The Royal College of Surgeons of England 1985.*

Drugs

Report of a working party on the use of controlled drugs in operating theatres. *The Association of Anaesthetists of Great Britain and Ireland 1981.*

Guidelines for safe and secure handling of medicines. A report to the Secretary of State for Social Services (Duthie Report). *Department of Health 1988.*

Examinations

Primary and final examinations for the FRCA: syllabus. *The Royal College of Anaesthetists March 1995.*

Intensive care

Adult intensive care report by a working group set up jointly by Clinical Resource and Audit Group (CRAG) and Scottish Health Management Efficiency Group. *Scottish Office Edinburgh 1992.*

Intensive care in the United Kingdom. *King's Fund Panel 1989* Anaesthesia *1989;* **44:** *428–431.*

Proposals for the content, assessment and organisation of training in intensive care medicine. *Intercollegiate Committee on Training in Intensive Care Medicine,* in press.

Standards for intensive care units. *Intensive Care Society 1985.*

Miscellaneous anaesthetic

Guidelines on duties of chairmen of divisions of anaesthesia. *Association of Anaesthetists of Great Britain and Ireland 1988.*

Report of the survey of anaesthetic practice. *The Association of Anaesthetists of Great Britain and Ireland 1988.*

Neurosurgery

Investigation into the neurosurgery patient transfers. *W. Wells, South Thames Regional Health Authority 1995.*

Report of the working party on the management of patients with serious head injury. *The Royal College of Surgeons of England 1988.*

NHS

Working for patients (White Paper). *Department of Health.*

Obstetrics

Anaesthetic facilities available at the place of birth. *National Birthday Trust 1986.*

Obstetric analgesia and anaesthesia in Scotland. *The National Medical Consultative Committee 1985.*

Personnel, hours

The new deal on junior doctors' hours El(91)82. *Department of Health.*

Implications for reductions in junior staff and the consultant-only hospital. *Association of Anaesthetists of Great Britain and Ireland.*

Purchasing

Guidance for purchasers. *The Royal College of Anaesthetists 1994.*

Quality

The A–Z of quality: a guide to quality initiatives in the NHS. *NHS Executive 1993.*

Research

Research for health – a research and development strategy for the NHS. *Department of Health.*

Resuscitation

Register of brain damage. Cardiac arrests report. *Quality of Practice Committee, Royal College of Anaesthetists.*

Training and education

A guide to specialist registrar training. *Department of Health.*

Faculty of anaesthetists: terms of reference for faculty tutors (March 1988). *The Royal College of Surgeons of England.*

Criteria for consultant status in anaesthesia. *The Royal College of Anaesthetists 1989.*

Faculty of anaesthetists: general professional training guide (June 1987). *The Royal College of Surgeons of England.*

Programme for identifying and training academic anaesthetists in the nineties. *The Royal College of Anaesthetists.*

Criteria for the staff anaesthetist grade. *The Royal College of Anaesthetists.*

A working paper on monitoring postgraduate and continuing medical and dental education. *The Standing Committee on Postgraduate Medical and Dental Education (SCOPME) September 1993.*

A good start: a report on job induction for hospital doctors and dentists in training. *The Standing Committee on Postgraduate Medical and Dental Education (SCOPME) November 1993.*

Teaching hospital doctors and dentists to teach. *Standing Committee on Postgraduate Medical and Dental Education (SCOPME) October 1994.*

A working paper on continuing professional development for doctors and dentists. *Standing Committee on Postgraduate Medical and Dental Education (SCOPME) September 1994.*

European specialist medical qualifications Order 1995; Statutory Instrument 1995 number 3208: *available from HMSO.*

Transplantation

Working Party on supply of donor organs for transplant. *Conference of Medical Royal Colleges in UK.*

Association of Anaesthetists of Great Britain and Ireland:
9 Bedford Square, London WC1B 3RA. Tel: 0171 631 1650

Audit Commission:
HMSO Publications Centre, PO Box 276, London SW8 5DT. Tel: 0171 873 9090

British Medical Association Joint Consultants Committee:
BMA House, Tavistock Square, London WC1H 9JP. Tel: 0171 387 4499

Caring for Children in the Health Services:
c/o NAWCH Ltd, Argyle House, 29–31 Euston Road, London NW1 2SD

Clinical Standards Advisory Group:
c/o HMSO Publications Centre, PO Box 276, London SW8 5DT. Tel: 0171 873 9090

Department of Health Research and Development Division:
Richmond House, 79 Whitehall, London SW1A 2NS

Department of Health:
DoH Mailings, c/o Two-Ten Communications Ltd, Building 150, Thorp Arch
Trading Estate, Wetherby, W. Yorkshire LS23 7EH. Tel: 01937 840250

Health Services Advisory Committee:
publications from HSE Books, PO Box 1999, Sudbury Suffolk CO10 6FS
Tel: 01787 881165.

HMSO Publications Centre, PO Box 276, London SW8 5DT. Tel: 0171 873 9090

Intercollegiate Committee on Training in Intensive Care Medicine:
c/o The Royal College of Anaesthetists

Joint Centre for Education in Medicine:
33 Millman Street, London WC1N 3EJ. Tel: 0171 831 6222

King's Fund:
11–13 Cavendish Square, London W1M 0AN. Tel: 0171 301 2400

London School of Hygiene and Tropical Medicine:
Keppel St, London WC1E 7HT. Tel: 0171 927 2339

Medical Defence Union Ltd, 3 Devonshire Place, London W1N 2EA

National Confidential Enquiry into Perioperative Deaths:
35-43 Lincoln's Inn Fields, London WC2A 3PN. Tel: 0171 831 6430

NHS Executive:
documents are available from Department of Health Mailings, or HMSO

Royal College of Anaesthetists:
48–49 Russell Square, London WC1B 4JY. Tel: 0171 813 1900

Royal College of Psychiatrists:
17 Belgrave Square, London SW1X 8PG. Tel: 0171 235 2351

Royal College of Surgeons of England:
Department of External Affairs, 35–43 Lincoln's Inn Fields, London WC2A 3PN.
Tel: 0171 405 3474, ext. 4173

Scottish Office:
Scottish Home and Health Department, St Andrew's House, Regent Rd, Edinburgh
EH1 3DE. Tel: 0131 556 8400

South Thames Regional Health Authority:
40 Eastbourne Terrace, London W2 3QR. Tel: 0171 725 2500

Standing Committee on Postgraduate Medical and Dental Education (SCOPME):
1 Park Square West, London NW1 4LJ. Tel: 0171 935 3916

The following is a list of all the safety notices issued by the Department of Health since December 1991 that have direct relevence to anaesthesia. Copies of individual notices can be obtained free of charge from the Medical Devices Agency, 0171 972 8225.

SN no.	Title	File no.	Date
SN 9702	Batteries used in critical care devices	9607300	Jan 97
SN 9638	Alton Dean pressure infusors: potential door failure	96100801	Dec 96
SN 9640	Infusion pumps: IVAC 770 syringe pumps: incorrect dose rate display	95110210	Dec 96
SN 9636	Demountable anaesthetic agent vaporizers	96092301	Nov 96
SN 9633	Syringe pump: Vickers Treonic IP3	96041501	Oct 96
SN 9630	Emergency resuscitation kit with pin-index regulator; Laerdal	96071503	Sept 96
SN 9628	Detatchable mains supply leads for use with medical devices. Reported problems	94032530	Sept 96
SN 9625	Infusion pump: IVAC P series pumps software upgrade	96052026	Aug 96
SN 9624	Lung ventilator: Ohmeda OAV7750: potential failure of power supply	95041304	Aug 96
SN 9622	Spacelabs ECG monitors software fault recall	96011910	Aug 96
SN 9621	Addendum to SN 9611 Graseby MS 2000 syringe pump: confusion over risk category	96022710	Aug 96
SN 9611	Graseby MS 2000 syringe pump: confusion over risk category	96022710	May 96
SN 9610	Pre-1989 Eschmann operation tables: potential failure of main hinge	95101216	March 96
SN 9609	Risk of skin burns from lead adaptors used with electrosurgical equipment	95110203	March 96
SN 9608	ARCP Medical Infusion Systems Ltd VP 5000 Series pumps: risk of electric shock from loose panel-mounted mains connector	95112706	March 96
SN 9607	Modification of Baxter Flo-Gard infusion pumps	95092607	March 96
SN 9606	Drager Oxylog ventilator pressure relief valve: risk of failure when autoclaved using the 134° Centigrade cycle	95021015	Feb 96

SN 9532	Marquette Responder 1200, 1250 and 1500 defibrillator: NiCd battery recall	95082111	Nov 95
SN 9531	Air flow incubators: risk of injury to babies when the airflow is inadvertently obstructed or diverted	95071213	Nov 95
SN 9528	Medix 2-pin universal mains leads: risk of electric shock	95072810	Oct 95
SN 9526	Greasebt Medical MS16A and MS26 ambulatory syringe pumps	95072502	Oct 95
SN 9517	Risk of burns to patients with attached monitoring lead, undergoing MRI scan	95020304	July 95
SN 9516	Decontamination of medical devices and equipment prior to investigation inspection, service or repair	95021502	July 95
SN 9509	Marquette Responder 1250 and 1500 Defibrillators: upgrade to prevent memory failure and device lockup	94092010	May 95
SN 9508	Possible detachment of heater grid from the Vickers combined infant radiant warmer/resuscitaire due to failure of retaining clips	95012405	May 95
SN 9506	Hydrophilic coated guide wires – stripping of coating: risk of embolism	94101107	April 95
SN 9506	Addendum to SAB(94)46 breathing system: hinged support arm failure	94060109	April 95
SN 9503	Risk of fire when using defibrillators in an oxygen-enriched atmosphere	94121309	Feb 95
SN 9502	Addendum to SAB(94)16 Becton Dickinson programme 1 and syringe pumps manufactured before 1990. Upgrade facility to high risk category requirements.	92040804	Feb 95
SN 9436	Hewlett Packard M11908 pulse oximeter adult finger probe: inappropriate use resulting in incorrect readings when used on paediatric patients	24/12/94031804	Sep 94
SN 9430	Cow & Gate 470 enteral feeding pump: change in delivery rate following momentary interruption of mains supply	28/03/10009	Aug 94
SN 9428	3M Defibrillator pads type 2345, 2346, 2345N and 2346N: manufacturer's recall	21/04/94021103	July 94
SN 9427	Welmed P1000, P2000 and P4000 syringe pumps: mandatory upgrade	28/01/94041922	July 94

SN 9426	Infusion pumps: incidents caused by fluid spillage and drop damage: should be checked by a qualified person	28/01/ 94010609	July 94
SN 9418	S&W Vickers DMS600 and DMS700 series defibrillators: modification to the carrying handle	21/04/ 93100714	May 94
SN 9413	Leakage of fresh gas from the medical gas supply hose via open flow control valves on the rotameters: follow up action	24/01/ 93110205	March 94
SN 9410	S&W Vickers Resuscitaires: defective pin-index yokes used for the location of gas cylinders	24/08/ 93102002	Feb 94
SN 9409	S&W Vickers Resuscitaire 165 flow meter control valve: over-tightening of valve knob may cause damage	24/08/ 92030403	Feb 94
SN 9408	Lifepak 10 defibrillator made by Phiso Control: manufacturer's modification	21/04/ 93102101	Feb 94
SN 9407	Vi-Tal Syringe pumps: withdrawal of technical support and spares	28/01/ 92100703	Feb 94
SN 9403	Cobe Laboratories Ltd Optima hollow fibre membrane oxygenators: possibility of air entering the arterial line	62/06/ 93110501	Jan 94
(94)01	Old style BOC oxygen regulators (part nos 350000 and 350140) possible fire hazard. These regulators are now obsolete and may not have been serviced by the manufacturer for some time	24/10/ 92101610	Jan 94
(93)63	Howorth Climator Mattress Heater Type PCM40: overheating	21/11/ 93052106	Dec 93
(93)60	Vial Medical SE Syringe pumps manufactured before 1986. May cease to infuse although continuing to indicate normal infusion	28/01/ 10162	Dec 93
(93)59	Pulse oximeter probes/transducers: risk of injury	24/12/ 93060211	Dec 93
(93)58	Puritan Bennett Cascade 1 Humidifiers: safety alert and addition of fire hazard labels	24/07/ 93101806	Dec 93
(93)57	Puritan Bennett Companion 2801 Portable ventilator: caution in using external battery	24/07/ 93062103	Dec 93

(93)52	Graseby 3300 PCA syringe pump: electrical interference may cause the pump to stop and revert to earlier infusion settings	28/01/ 93073013	Dec 93
(93)51	Infusion pump mains connectors: ingress of leaked fluids	28/01/ 93052107	Nov 93
(93)50	Laerdal Silicone Resuscitators: inadvertant positive end expiratory pressure (PEEP)	24/08/ 93081307	Nov 93
(93)44	Care of the Intavent Ltd Laryngeal mask. New guidelines for their care	66/03/ 92031709	Sept 93
(93)42	Kendall Curity 8.5 mm tracheal tubes quarantined in accordance with hazard notice (93)23	66/01/930 61717	Sept 93
(93)41	Mercury contamination of baby incubators: the need for vigilance	25/01/ 93061603	Sept 93
(93)37	Degradation of plastic i.v. catheters with interactions with solvent-based spray dressings and disinfectants	62/13/ 93063002	Sept 93
(93)35	Draeger 4200 babytherm infant radiant warmer: security of warmer bearing assembly	25/01/ 91112521	Aug 93
(93)34	HG Wallace Ltd – i.v. cannulae code 519 16G labelling error batch 211292: recall	62/139306 2203	Aug 93
(93)33	Graseby MS2000 syringe pump: displayed preset volume may differ from the actual volume to be infused	28/01/ 93042303	July 93
(93)30	Gas supply tubing to nebulizers: incorrect selection for use	24/14/ 92091103	July 93
(93)27	Syringe pumps: uncontrolled infusion	28/01/ 92060207	June 93
(93)26	Ohmeda OAC 7700 ventilator: air entrainment caused patient awareness	24/07/ 93041307	June 93
(93)22	IVAC model 560/565 volumetric infusion pump sets, codes G52503, 52100, G52703: leak at pressure-sensing disc	62/01/ 92061812	May 93
(93)16	Carbon dioxide cylinders: inappropriate use	54/09/ 92120703	March 93
(93)04	Simed S100 pulse oximeters: risk of battery overheating	24/12/ 10029	Jan 93
(92)55	Anaesthetic machines: Ohmeda vaporizer compatibility blocks	24/01/ 92041602	Oct 92

(92)49	United States Food & Drug Administration withdrawal of approval for smallbore catheters used in continuous spinal anaesthesia	68/03 92050604	Sept 92
(92)31	Tycos pressure infusor model 5099-01: risk of failure, product to be withdrawn or regularly inspected	28/01 10085	April 92
(92)30	Suction equipment for use with piped medical gas system: malfunction of safety devices	24/11 10048	April 92
(92)29	Anaesthetic agent vaporizers fitted with agent-specific fillers: reports of overfilling	24/02/ 92010202	April 92
(92)13	Heated humidifiers: correct positioning and security of temperature-monitoring probes	24/03/ 91111115	Feb 92
(92)12	Heated humidifiers when used with lung ventilators: risk of excessive temperature	24/03/ 10005	Feb 92
(92)03	Ohmeda adjustable pressure-limiting valves: risk of failure	24/11/ 10048	Jan 92

Index